BREEDING
from your BITCH

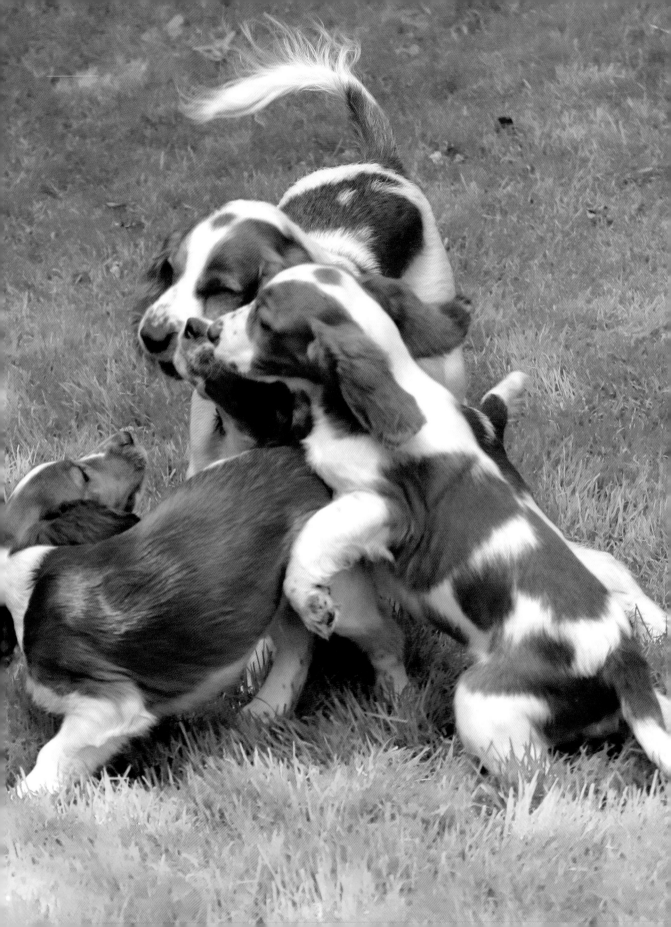

BREEDING
from your
BITCH

Tony Buckwell

THE CROWOOD PRESS

First published in 2019 by
The Crowood Press Ltd
Ramsbury, Marlborough
Wiltshire SN8 2HR

www.crowood.com

British Library Cataloguing-in-Publication Data
A catalogue record for this book is available from the British Library.

ISBN 978 1 78500 653 1

Acknowledgements
I could not have written or illustrated this book without the
encouragement, guidance and assistance of many people. I would
particularly wish to acknowledge the expertise, advice and support of my
wife, Wendy, without which I would have been unable to undertake the
task. I should also wish to thank Mrs Diane Stevens who generously enabled
me to photograph her dogs being used at stud, and express my gratitude to
my many friends in the South Eastern Gundog Society and the Kent & East
Sussex branch of the Utility Gundog Society. Last but by no means least, my
special thanks to Angela Gilchrist, the consultant clinical psychologist who
first encouraged me to take up writing to help overcome the devastating
effects of clinical depression.

Typeset by Jean Cussons Typesetting, Diss, Norfolk

Printed and bound in India by Parksons Graphics

CONTENTS

INTRODUCTION

It can be very rewarding to breed from your bitch but this is not a matter to be undertaken lightly. Whilst, in principle, anyone can breed from their dog, whether they should or not is another matter entirely. There are people who will point out the number of unwanted dogs in rehoming centres and claim that breeding further puppies simply adds to the problem. There will be others who believe everyone has the right and that most bitches benefit from having a litter. The moderate view to which most in society would seem to subscribe is that only 'responsible breeders' should be producing puppies; people who know what they are doing, take great care to provide for the welfare of their dogs, produce healthy puppies of good temperament and make every attempt to ensure their puppies only go to suitable homes.

1 DECIDING TO BREED FROM YOUR BITCH

The decision to breed from your bitch requires careful consideration and forward planning. Before deciding, you need to be aware of and weigh up all the pros and cons of dog breeding.

In the first instance, before making any decision on whether or not to breed from a bitch, it will be worth asking yourself the following questions:

- Is my bitch fit and healthy and does she have a good temperament? Do I know what health testing is recommended in the breed and can I afford to pay for any necessary prior health testing?
- Can I afford to pay for a caesarean operation should it be necessary?
- Can I cope with a large litter of, say, eight to ten puppies? Have I the time to devote to rearing the puppies until they are ready to go? Have I the space to provide a suitable area for the bitch to whelp and then to house and socialize older energetic puppies?

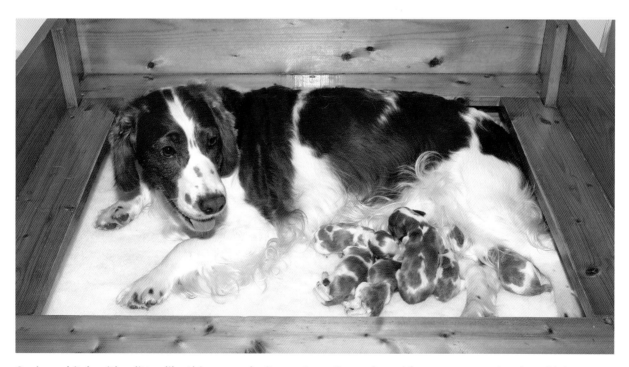

Seeing a bitch with a litter like this can make it very tempting to breed from your own dog, but think very carefully and weigh up all the pros and cons associated with raising a litter of puppies before deciding on a mating.

- Do I know enough about all that's involved in breeding and raising a litter? Will I be able to help the bitch through whelping, or can I confidently rely on someone to help me? Do I know how to rear the puppies including their appropriate worming, vaccination and socialization and can I advise their new owners on how best to feed, rear and train them?
- Am I reasonably likely to find good homes for the puppies? There are certain times of the year when it is more difficult to sell puppies, for example either when people are away on holiday or during the colder winter months.
- Am I able to take back or rehome a puppy if it were to become necessary?

Only when you are in a position to answer 'yes' to each of these questions should you contemplate breeding a litter of puppies.

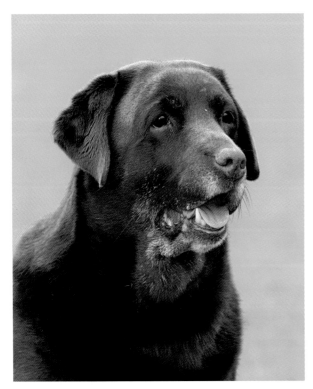

Mature bitches will often show accelerated signs of ageing after having had a litter.

It has been estimated that some 10,000 unwanted dogs have to be euthanized by local authorities in the UK each year and around a quarter of that number, both pedigree and cross-breeds, are held in rescue centres awaiting new homes. You must have convincing reasons to breed from your dog since otherwise you might potentially be adding to that surplus. Ask yourself the question, 'Why am I breeding from my dog?' Make sure you are entering this process with no misapprehensions of the claimed advantages of letting your bitch have a litter of puppies and are fully aware of the potential consequences should anything go wrong.

There are a number of popular myths used by owners to justify breeding from their pet bitch and we will be exploring some of these in the following sections. Certainly, if you are breeding with the intention of keeping a puppy, do make sure the mating you plan is likely to produce the puppy you want, aware of the fact that the puppy you require might more likely be secured (at considerably less cost) from a reputable, experienced breeder who has puppies available for sale that are of a suitable type.

POPULAR MYTHS

It will be good for the bitch

Whilst it is true that the incidence of pyometra or endometrial hypoplasia (a disease in which pus accumulates in the uterus – the bitch's womb) is lower among multiparous bitches (those that have had a number of litters), there is no evidence to indicate that having one or two litters of puppies has any positive welfare benefit for a bitch.

However, there are many reasons to suggest that being bred can prove detrimental to a bitch.

Dogs will occasionally show accelerated signs of ageing after having a litter. Not all bitches are good mothers. Some can become distressed and either ignore or savage their pups; others can be clumsy mothers, a particular problem among some of the physically larger breeds, and will lie on and crush their puppies causing them to suffocate. Bitches can have severe delivery problems and even die in the process, although the latter is

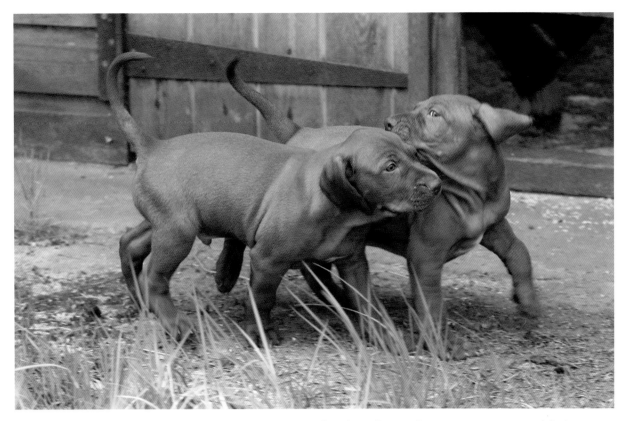

A pair of boisterous Vizsla puppies playing together. Before breeding make sure you can cope with the challenges of raising a litter of active puppies, particularly as they get older and demand suitable space and sufficient resources to meet their requirements.

relatively uncommon provided they are afforded prompt veterinary attention.

A bitch should have a litter before being spayed
There is no reason for a bitch to have had a litter before being spayed. Whilst there may be certain disadvantages to spaying very young, immature bitches (notably an increased risk of incontinence associated with altered hormone levels following spaying) there is no physical advantage for a bitch to have been pregnant and raised puppies before being spayed.

It will be good for the children
There is no doubt that it can be highly beneficial for children to experience the pleasure of seeing new life born and be introduced to the

chores and responsibilities associated with having to care for young animals. Unfortunately life is not always straightforward and complications can arise. One or more puppies may be stillborn and others may die within the first few days of life. These events are likely to be emotionally distressing and only you can judge the likely effect it might have on your children. Most whelping takes place in the early hours when children are most likely to want to sleep and otherwise be tired and irritable – extremely distracting when you are wanting to give your dog your undivided attention. If the bitch should need a caesarean, this is likely to entail a rush to the vet at times when child minders are rarely available at such necessary short notice. A healthy litter will take up a great deal of your time and sap your energy for several weeks. Hand-rearing puppies will be even more exhausting and caring for sick puppies can prove distressing. Young children are hardly likely to benefit from the reduced level of attention or your increased stress levels on these occasions.

It will calm her down

There is absolutely no scientific evidence to suggest that having a litter of puppies has any influence on a bitch's temperament. Many dogs show a tendency to become calmer with increasing age and maturity but this is just as true for male dogs as for bitches, and in bitches that have never had a litter. Any apparent calming effect associated with pregnancy and lactation is purely coincidental and likely to be a temporary change associated with the bitch's preoccupation with the process of pregnancy and nursing her puppies.

Temperament is dependent on a variety of factors, particularly genetic (dogs can inherit behavioural traits from their parents), management (the way in which you raise and train your dog), environmental and also how mature she may be at the time.

A further consideration should be the fact that bitches that are hyperactive and excitable whilst pregnant and lactating are likely to pass the trait on to their offspring. They are likely to be no different afterwards and all you will succeed in doing is thereby perpetuating the problem.

You are more likely to succeed in reducing a dog's boisterous and excitable behaviour by enlisting the help of a reputable dog trainer and/ or behavioural counsellor than you are from letting her have a litter of puppies.

I will be able to keep a puppy that is just like my bitch

If you really want another dog that will, as far as possible, replicate the characteristics and features of your bitch, then you are likely to be disappointed if you plan on breeding from her and keeping a puppy. This is because the pups will share genes (the molecular units of heredity)

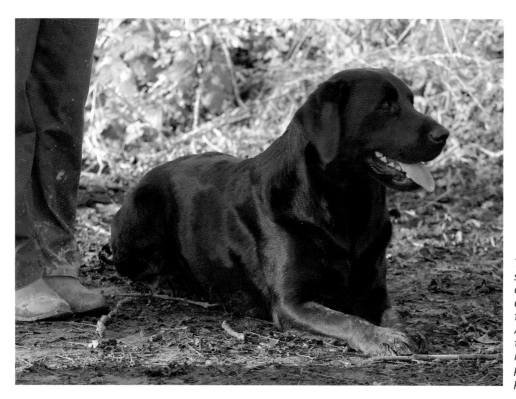

Temperament should be a prime consideration in deciding to breed from your dog. A calm, steady temperament is likely to be passed on to the puppies.

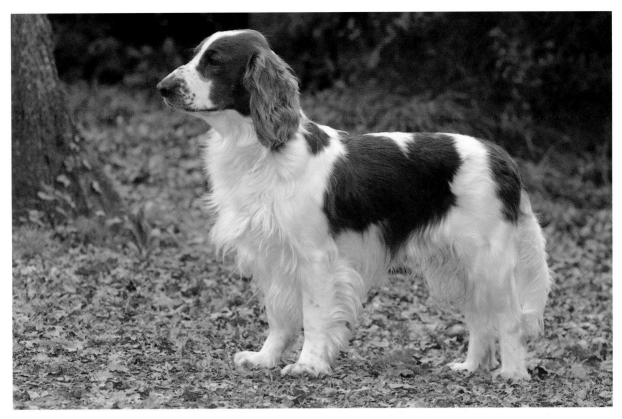

Ideally select a stud dog that has been health tested and found to have satisfactory results, that is known to pass on characteristics you desire and with a genetic background that complements that of your bitch.

from both the sire and the dam and there is no guarantee whatsoever that they will necessarily inherit the best features of both.

Breeding to a stud dog without a clear understanding of his genetic background is almost certainly likely to produce disappointing results. Without knowing something of the sire's prior performance at stud your puppies could potentially inherit all of his worst points and none of your bitch's good points.

The most likely means of getting another dog that is similar to yours is by acquiring a sibling, either a brother or sister from the same litter, or a puppy from a litter produced by repeat mating her parents.

To make money

Although they won't always admit to it, this is certainly one element that often motivates people when they decide to breed a litter of puppies. It is very tempting, knowing the price people will expect to pay for a puppy, to multiply that figure by six or more and assume there is a nice little profit to be made in dog breeding. Unfortunately life isn't always quite so simple and responsible dog breeding, particularly from pedigree dogs, is a costly exercise – one where you can all too easily find yourself significantly out of pocket.

Whilst it is certainly true that some people make money out of breeding dogs, these will be people who regularly breed dogs of a type that are relatively easy to sell. At the extreme end of the market, profits from puppy farming come at the cost of the animals' welfare. The situation for someone breeding responsibly, producing one or two litters from a pet bitch, can be entirely different.

THE COSTS INVOLVED

There are a variety of costs that should be taken into account when breeding from your bitch for the first time. Assuming she is a pedigree dog, registered with the Kennel Club, and you wish to register her puppies, the likely expenses that you might reasonably expect to incur will include the cost of:

- The stud fee (typically equivalent to the cost of a puppy)
- Any necessary veterinary health testing (for inherited and other breed-predisposed conditions)
- Worming and veterinary antenatal care for your bitch
- The extra food required during pregnancy and whilst the bitch is lactating
- An appropriate whelping box and plenty of soft, washable veterinary bedding
- An infrared heat lamp and/or heated pads for pups to cuddle up, especially at times when their dam is not with them
- Worming the puppies and your lactating bitch
- Kennel Club registration for each puppy
- Food for the puppies after weaning
- Any advertising costs
- Microchipping, preliminary vaccination and veterinary checks on puppies prior to sale
- Cost(s) of the extra care and vaccinations for any pups unsold after eight weeks.

In addition, a contingency fund must be available to cover the cost of an emergency out-of-hours caesarean operation and any other emergency postnatal care that may be required by your lactating bitch or her puppies.

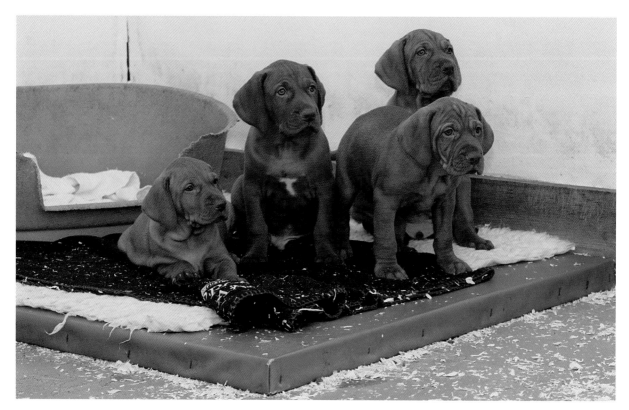

Do not underestimate the costs involved in breeding and raising a litter of puppies like these Hungarian Vizslas. Try to realistically budget for the financial costs, including a suitable allowance for any likely contingencies.

Depending on your circumstances, you might also need to take into consideration the possibility of having to take unpaid leave from work should you need to be with the puppies at any time.

The cost to you

The true cost of breeding a litter, of course, is more than financial.

The greater cost is the physical and mental effort you will have to put into the exercise, even if everything goes smoothly and according to plan. Don't underestimate the additional stress and strain that you will find yourself having to bear if anything should go wrong. It will be very distressing if you find your bitch requires emergency medical attention, or if the puppies become sick, especially if some should die, or if you are left with unsold puppies.

Probably the two most personally challenging aspects of breeding a litter of puppies, however, will be the time involved and the associated mess that you will need to clear up.

The time and mess factors

A pregnant bitch requires your absolute and undivided attention throughout parturition, during the whole time from when she first shows signs of going into labour until several hours after her last puppy is born and successfully suckling. This whole process can take at least twenty-four to thirty-six hours, usually longer, meaning you will be getting very little sleep during this period.

Thereafter a responsible adult needs to be on the premises at all times, able to attend to the bitch and her puppies for the next seven to eight weeks.

Ensuring that puppies are kept clean, fed and generally well cared for is an enormously time-consuming business.

When they are weaned you will be feeding the puppies at least four meals a day. The number of meals fed at this time will primarily depend on the breed of dog (smaller puppies tend to be given smaller meals, more frequently) and whether the bitch continues to suckle the pups or you remove her entirely.

This is only part of your responsibilities. Most bitches make a good job of cleaning up after their pups; at least they do until the pups start to be weaned at around three weeks of age.

Everything changes at weaning.

From this time onwards, the bitch will cease cleaning up after her puppies; this becomes your job. As fast as you clean them up, they will get messy again. The cleaning-up process takes place every time you feed (four to six times daily), and in-between where necessary. This process is no fun at all and only seems to get worse; the bigger and livelier the puppies, the less fun and more challenging the cleaning process. You will need a mountain of newspaper and what will seem like a lake of disinfectant and detergent. You will require endless patience and limitless endurance because just when all seems clean and tidy at last, you will likely have to get right up and start all over again.

This is hard and smelly work.

IS DOG BREEDING WORTH ALL THE TIME AND EFFORT REQUIRED?

Assuming your dog is fit, healthy and of a suitable temperament, there is no doubt that it is extremely satisfying, having taken the trouble to select a suitable stud, to breed puppies that are likely to improve on the qualities that your bitch already displays and, potentially, pass on those characteristics to future generations.

The primary reason for many people to breed dogs is to keep a puppy and in doing so improve on the qualities displayed by their dog or dogs. If you either exhibit your dog in the show ring and/or compete in working tests and field trials, it can be even more rewarding if either your puppy or another from the same litter excels in either discipline.

Furthermore, if the breed is rare, by carefully selecting a suitable stud dog you can help to further improve and propagate the breed.

Dog breeding is psychologically and emotionally rewarding. Pets can greatly influence how we feel about ourselves, and life in general. They are 'teachers and healers of extraordinary talent'. Research shows that pet owners have

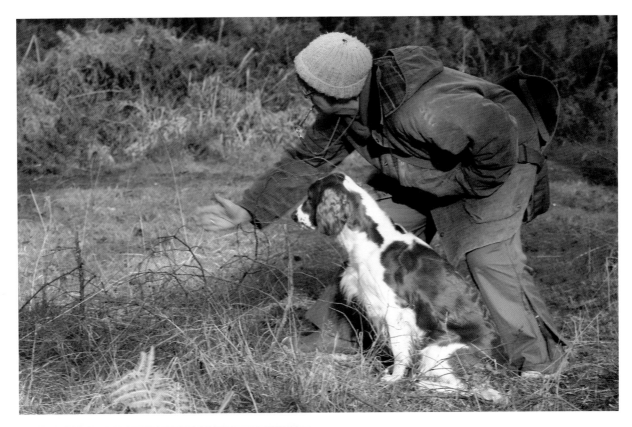

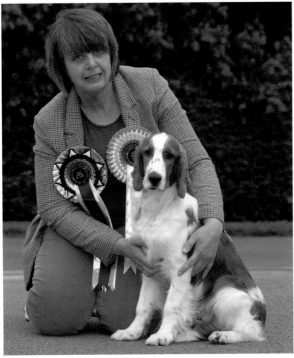

Top and left: *Research shows that dog ownership is good for people, and breeding a puppy that you can successfully train to work in the field or go on to successfully compete in the show ring will further provide immense satisfaction.*

greater self-esteem, are more physically fit, tend to be less lonely, are more conscientious, more extraverted, and tend to be less fearful and less preoccupied than non-owners.

Everyone needs to feel needed and have something to care for and pet ownership can be a very effective means of satisfying that need. Families surveyed before and after they acquired a pet reported feeling happier after adding a pet to the family. So extending your experience of pet ownership by breeding suitable puppies that in appropriate homes are likely to further enrich the lives of other people, will in itself be an extremely rewarding experience.

It is also very satisfying to learn how well your puppies are doing in their new homes and to find how content their new owners are with their progress and how they are turning into valued companions either around the home or, if it's to be a working dog, around the farm or on the shooting field. Dog owners generally have been shown to have more and better social interactions and many dog breeders will tell you how some of their new puppy owners have subsequently become life-long friends.

Finally, of course, if all goes well you may even be able to make a modest amount of money from the sale of the litter.

2 PLANNING A LITTER, MATING AND CONFIRMING PREGNANCY

So you have read the first chapter, and been able to answer 'yes' to all of the questions. You have decided that you are thinking of breeding puppies for good reasons and are determined to go ahead; what initial steps do you need to take?

FORWARD PLANNING

It is useful to plan ahead with some realistic understanding of the necessary timescales. Waiting until your bitch is in season and ready to be mated before selecting the stud dog and arranging the mating is unlikely to achieve optimum success. However, by understanding the overall process and estimating how long each step will take, you will be able to plan ahead and anticipate any potential problems.

Forward planning will ensure that your bitch won't whelp when it's least convenient or you won't have a large litter ready to go at times when people are least likely to want to take on and train a new puppy. Forward planning is also essential to ensure that the pups will be raised in the most appropriate environment, that the bitch is fully vaccinated, up to date with her vaccinations and wormed prior to mating and again before whelping.

The preparatory phase, selecting the stud dog and having all necessary health checks carried out (outlined in this chapter) should be undertaken well in advance of any intended

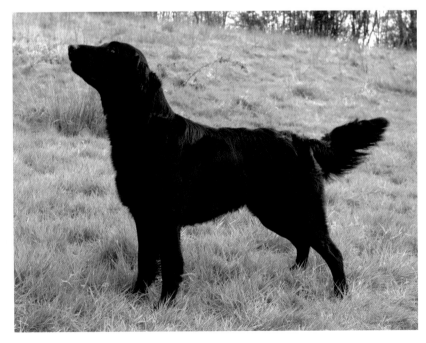

It is important to understand your bitch's strengths and weaknesses; her good and bad points. Try to get an informed opinion from a reputable breeder and take advice concerning a suitable stud dog that will complement her good points and/or compensate for any weaknesses.

litter; certainly nine to twelve months in advance of mating your bitch.

CHOOSING A STUD DOG

Finding a stud dog is a fairly fundamental requirement. A careful choice of stud dog will be essential. No doubt the process of selecting a suitable dog from the many that may potentially be available would appear to be a daunting task and whilst in many respects this is true, there are certain points to bear in mind that, when taken together, will help narrow the choice considerably.

Do your homework

Learn about any problems that are within your breed (such as hip dysplasia [HD], progressive retinal atrophy [PRA], and so on). Do as much research as you can to learn about any inherited traits you are hoping to change. Should any of your bitch's unwanted traits be inherited, you do not want to use a stud dog that may also have the trait and therefore not be able to correct it.

In order to gauge the risks of a stud dog carrying a recessive gene, you would need to examine the stud dog's ancestry; its pedigree. When it's an unwanted trait that is inherited polygenically (caused by several genes when combined together), it would depend on how badly the stud dog is affected as to the outcome of the pups not inheriting the gene and the best way to establish this would be to check out the stud dog's siblings.

Know your bitch – her strengths and weaknesses

Be honest with yourself and be as objective as you can when it comes to assessing your bitch's strengths and weak points. Know what's important and prioritize which traits you consider to be good, and which you would like to pass on in her pups.

Get an honest opinion of your bitch from a few breeders. Find out what they think; what do they consider to be her virtues and which are her faults. Get several breeders' opinions of a good choice for a stud dog that will enhance your bitch's strengths and correct any particular weak-

nesses. Your aim should be to use the dog that is most likely to correct any of her weaknesses and seek to avoid one that will undermine or dilute any of her good points.

You have to bear in mind that the chances of finding a stud dog that complements your bitch 100 per cent are low, so it is far better to focus on her weaker traits when looking for a stud dog. Certainly it will be important to find a dog that does not share her faults because, ideally, you will be seeking a stud dog that has a track record of correcting such weaknesses in the breed.

Health issues, soundness and temperament

Ideally both bitch and dog will be fully health tested so that you can be confident that in breeding, you are unlikely to pass on any inherited problems to the puppies.

Ask your vet to perform a physical examination and give advice regarding your bitch's suitability for breeding. Most bitches should be at least a year old before mating and have had at least one normal season. It's usually advisable, however, to breed from her a little later, once she's fully mature, typically after she has had at least three to four normal seasons. Usually this will mean she is between three to six years of age. It is not advisable to start breeding an older bitch and certainly not beyond the age of eight. Knowing she cycles regularly will help you anticipate when she is likely to come into season, at what time she will be ready for mating, and when any puppies will be due to go to new homes.

Health testing will represent a financial commitment so take strategic advice and decide which tests to have carried out first. There is no point carrying out some blood tests to confirm the bitch is clear of a number of relatively rare conditions in the breed only to subsequently find she shows signs of a more common debilitating condition, such as hip dysplasia.

Once you know the bitch's health status and suitability for breeding you will be in a better position to assess the comparative health status of potential stud dogs. Assuming the stud dog owners have undertaken health testing, ask to see copies of the results, don't simply take their word for it. If you have done your homework and understand any health issues in the breed, see how familiar an owner is with these problems and how they compare their dogs in these respects. You should find that most reputable breeders will be very well informed, a 'font of knowledge', and in speaking with them your understanding of the health of the breed will improve considerably.

Stud dog owners who are members of the Kennel Club Assured Breeder Scheme undertake to carry out health testing of all their breed stock, will give you good advice and assistance, and will often take an interest in finding good homes for your puppies.

Aim to breed a litter that will represent an improvement on the parents

Resist the temptation to breed thinking you are likely to simply reproduce your bitch. Remember the stud dog will contribute equally to the characteristics of the puppies. The intention in breeding should be to improve on the dog you already own so identify the characteristics that you would wish to improve upon and then try to select a stud dog accordingly. Don't necessarily select a stud simply because it happens to be in your locality and it is convenient. Try to use a proven stud dog wherever possible, preferably one owned by a reputable breeder and trainer who should be able to show you progeny of the 'type' you are seeking.

Don't focus on just one line

It's far better to keep your options open and judge your choice as objectively as you possibly can than arbitrarily selecting a well-known kennel from which to choose a stud dog. If a par-

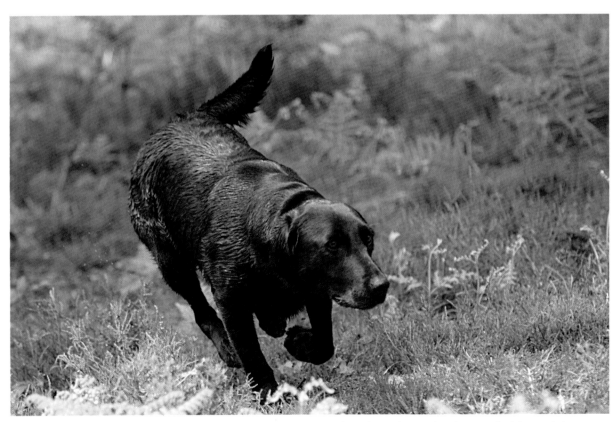

It is essential to take temperament and soundness into consideration when selecting a suitable stud dog. These are important traits that you will aim to pass on to your puppies.

ticular stud dog will match your bitch and help strengthen her good points and/or eliminate any weak traits, then you should consider that dog as an option to use.

Check the coefficient of inbreeding

Inbreeding, the continuous mating of closely related individuals over successive generations, will have a detrimental influence on health. The coefficient of inbreeding (COI) indicates how genetically similar the offspring of a mating are. There are online programmes you can use to calculate the COI of every proposed pedigree, and some of these programmes, such as the UK Kennel Club's 'Mate-Select', are free. This is a very good way of estimating how inbred any puppies you breed would actually be, which in turn helps calculate the risk of their inheriting recessive traits. You stand a much better chance of breeding healthier pups using matings with lower COIs because hereditary health issues are usually inherited recessively.

Calculate the COI that will result from breeding your bitch to each of the stud dogs that you are interested in using. The smaller the COI, and especially if the percentage is under 10 per cent, the better. If this is the case, you should definitely add the dog to your list of potential studs.

Never, however, become too preoccupied with any one particular criteria when selecting your stud dog. Remember that tools like COIs and EBVs (estimated breeder values) are available to assist in selecting the best dog to use; they should not be relied upon to solely dictate which particular dog to choose.

Temperament and soundness

Ideally you will want to use a healthy stud dog with a proven track record of producing sound puppies. Go to see as many of the stud dogs and their offspring as you can. You may instinctively feel it would be best to use a champion dog simply because he is a good representative of his breeds; however, a top show breeder once pointed out that, unless you are in a position to evaluate his progeny, the stud dog that produced that champion may be a better choice to sire successful puppies.

Temperament is dependent on a variety of factors, particularly genetic, environmental and management factors (the way in which you raise and train your dog) as well as how mature she may be. Good dog breeders will say, quite rightly, that the temperament of both sire and dam should be a prime consideration when deciding whether or not to breed from a dog. Temperament is inherited notwithstanding the fact that environmental factors – in particular the way a puppy is raised and trained – will have a significant influence on the dog's subsequent behaviour.

Consider using a sire that is not over-used

Using a dog that is extremely popular might be tempting. However, it is important to consider the effect on the breed as a whole. If a stud dog is used on a significant proportion of the available bitches, particularly in numerically small breeds, it will reduce the size of the gene pool available from which to select further, future matings. Consequently there is a risk of creating a 'genetic bottleneck' making it harder in future to find a stud dog that boasts a different set of complementary traits.

Consider using an older rather than a younger stud dog

It's worth using an older dog because they will have reached maturity and any inherited age-related health issues will have manifested themselves, whereas in a younger dog, the chances are they have not. Another advantage is that an older dog is likely to have sired previous litters, meaning that there will be more examples of his progeny available for you to assess. A potential disadvantage of using an older dog is that the sperm count (the overall number of viable sperm as a proportion of each ejaculate) tends to decline as dogs get older and become more senile.

Location

Whilst you should not choose a stud dog purely because it is conveniently close to home, you should choose to take your bitch to a stud that's not too far away from where you live. This makes life a whole lot easier if you find you have to have your bitch mated at relatively short notice, as

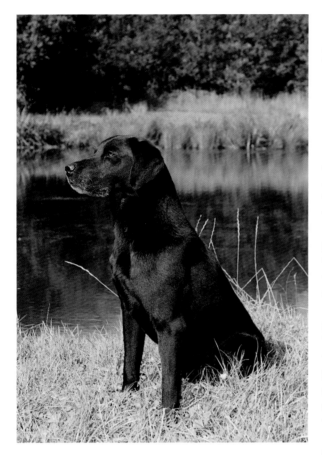

Consider using an older stud dog and proven sire like this Field Champion Labrador. There is likely to be progeny from previous litters he has sired that you can assess.

well as reducing the cost of all the travelling you may have to do.

HEALTH TESTING

The purpose of health testing is to attempt to identify and, where possible, control disease both within the individual affected dog and, when the dog is to be used for breeding, within the breed population as a whole. There are various forms of health tests and the type of test used is largely dependent on the type and character of the disease to be identified.

In this context it is important to understand and distinguish between the terms phenotype and genotype. A dog's phenotype relates to its outward appearance in all of its anatomical, physiological and behavioural characteristics. The phenotype may be influenced not only by the genetic make-up of the dog, but also by physical and environmental factors, such as the amount, type and frequency of exercise it receives, the type and quantity of food it is fed and so on.

The genotype refers to the entire genetic constitution of an individual and is determined by the genes it inherits from the parents. The genotype is unaffected by any other intrinsic or external environmental factors.

Phenotypic tests
Traditionally vets have had to rely on examining the phenotype to determine the presence and severity of inherited diseases. These are clinical tests that seek to identify and in some cases classify specific characteristic signs of the disease that can be observed in affected individuals.

Using these tests a variety of formal testing schemes have been devised and applied that have helped breeders reduce the incidence and/or severity of the disease in the breed population, and owners to understand how best to try to ameliorate the signs of the disease should their dog be affected. Examples include:

The BVA/KC hip scoring scheme whereby dogs' hips are X-rayed and the radiographs are submitted for examination by a panel of formally appointed experts who score the hips according to agreed criteria. Each hip is evaluated by two experts who score nine anatomical features and score each hip out of a total of 53. The two scores are then added together to give an overall total hip score. So, a dog's hip score can range from 0 to 106, and the lower the hip scores, the better the anatomy of the dog's hips.

In breeds where significant numbers of dogs have been through the hip scheme, it is possible to calculate a breed mean hip score, which gives a feel for the average score within that breed.

For the purpose of the BVA/KC hip scoring scheme, a dog has to be positioned carefully. Here the dog is lying in a frame that ensures the chest is upright and the pelvis is level. The hind legs are extended and taped together to ensure that the radiographic image of the hip joint can be properly evaluated and correctly scored.

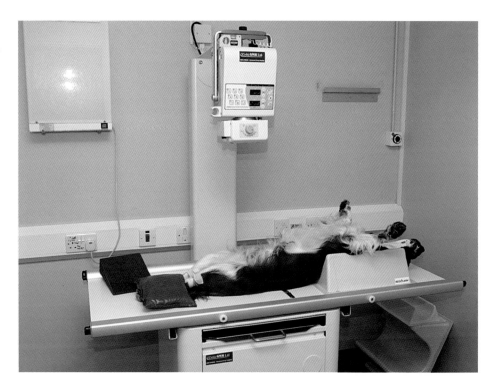

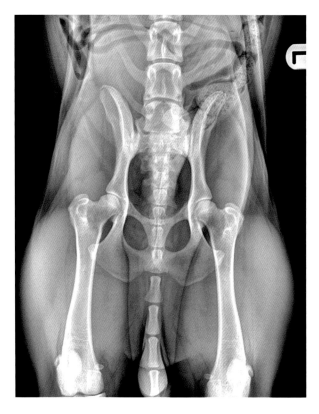

A hip X-ray taken for the purpose of the BVA/KC hip scoring scheme. Radiographs submitted for evaluation must include the dog's unique KC registration number and microchip number; for reasons of confidentiality these have been deleted from this particular image.

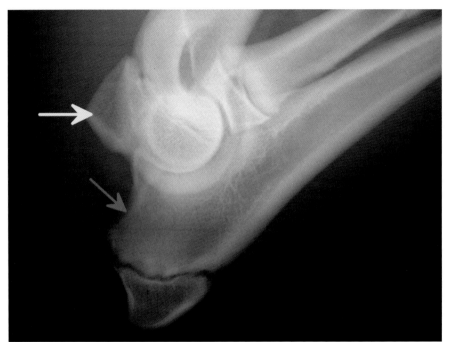

An X-ray photograph illustrating an un-united anconeal process (white arrow). This represents a gross form of elbow dysplasia and affected dogs will be unsuitable for breeding. The red arrow shows where the anconeal process should normally attach. (Photo: Dr Gary Clayton-Jones)

The X-ray appearance and scheme score can thus be used to help select less severely affected dogs for breeding.

The BVA/KC elbow grading scheme is similarly applied to X-rays taken of the dogs' elbows. In this case the X-ray appearance of each elbow is graded by two panel specialists from 0–3 depending on certain observable criteria; the lower the grade, the better the anatomy of the elbow. In this scheme, if the dog has two different elbow grades, the higher of the two is used as the dog's elbow grade.

Breeders are advised to use only unaffected dogs for breeding and the grade will usually determine if an individual dog is likely to subsequently become lame as a result of elbow dysplasia. Surgery to ameliorate the signs of disease can also be attempted in higher graded dogs. The grading scheme is helpful to owners and breeders alike. Not only will it determine if a dog is suitable for breeding but the result obtained is likely to determine if an individual dog is likely to require subsequent veterinary treatment or, if suitable for work, warrants investment in the time and cost of training.

The BVA/KC/ISDS (International Sheep Dog Society) eye scheme requires dogs to be examined by a member of a specialist panel of veterinary ophthalmologists who examine their eyes, looking for characteristic signs of breed-specific inherited eye conditions. These conditions are categorized as two lists: Schedule A conditions and Schedule B conditions. Schedule A contains all of the known inherited eye diseases and the breeds that are currently known to be affected by these conditions. Schedule B lists breeds and conditions where further investigation is urged. Specialist panellists, appointed by the BVA, can examine any individual dog for clinical signs of these diseases. Unfortunately many of these inherited eye diseases are not present from birth and breeders especially are advised to have their breeding stock examined throughout their dog's life.

DNA testing

A gene is the basic physical and functional unit of heredity. Genes are made up of DNA (deoxyribonucleic acid). DNA has a complex double-helix structure rather like a coiled ladder that is able

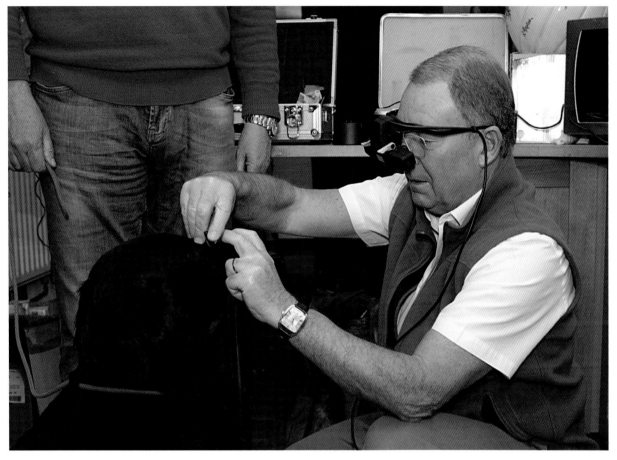

One of the specialist veterinary ophthalmologists appointed by the BVA examines a dog for the purpose of the BVA/KC/ISDS eye scheme.

to replicate itself. A gene is simply a small part of this complex double helical structure.

By comparing the DNA from dogs affected by a genetic disorder with DNA from normal individuals, the difference (the defective gene) can be established and analysed. A DNA test can then be developed that identifies other cells that have that same defective gene. Since those cells will each have two copies, one inherited from each parent, the DNA test will also determine whether one or both copies are defective.

DNA tests look at the dog's genotype as distinct from its phenotype. They tell us whether the dog has inherited a genetic condition and the likelihood of passing that condition on to any progeny.

To submit material for DNA testing we usually collect either a small blood sample or a buccal swab (a sample of cells taken on a small brush rubbed just inside the cheek). Samples are sent to a reference laboratory, often the laboratory that first developed the test. Testing typically takes about a week.

DNA tests are only available for a limited number of diseases and a DNA test will only reveal information about the particular disease being tested for, not each and every inherited condition. Nevertheless more and more DNA tests are continually being developed. Information on the tests that are available for particular breeds can be found online via the Kennel Club's Breed Information Centre, or by contacting the relevant breed club, your veterinary surgeon and/or your dog's breeder.

The benefits of health testing

The results of health testing are valuable to owners and breeders alike. Knowing your dog has an inherited disorder, you are able to make informed decisions; for example, on how much exercise to give it, what to feed it, whether it is suitable for breeding and if so what type of dog to mate it to, and of course whether or not it is likely to require veterinary drug treatment or surgical intervention to alleviate the signs of the disease. Significant progress is now being made in developing a variety of tools that used intelligently, can assist breeders increase the likelihood of producing healthy puppies.

Despite the fact that the BVA/KC schemes have rarely eliminated hereditary conditions, over the years they have generally reduced the incidence and overall severity of a number of serious breed-predisposed conditions.

The hip and elbow schemes were quite ambitious in attempting to address what we now understand are two quite complex inherited orthopaedic conditions. Hip and elbow dysplasia are likely to be polygenic (caused by more than one gene acting together) and influenced by a variety of extrinsic factors such as diet and exercise. Nevertheless using test results for hip dysplasia and knowing the genealogy of closely-related dogs in these respects, in other words knowing the scores of parents and other closely related dogs, statistical analyses can now be made to determine the likelihood of an individual dog passing on the condition to its progeny.

The results of these analyses, called EBVs (estimated breeder values), are now published by the UK Kennel Club for KC registered dogs and are freely available online via the Mate Select programme. Mate Select also allows you to calculate the degree of inbreeding, or coefficient of inbreeding (COI), for potential puppies that could be produced from a hypothetical mating.

EBVs have been successfully applied for many years in improving production among food-producing farmed livestock and we have every hope that similar use can be made to improve pedigree dogs. EBVs are only available for breeds with a large number and wide spread of tested dogs. The more dogs there are that have been scored in a dog's pedigree, the greater the confidence in the accuracy of the EBV. Consequently it is now, more than ever, important that owners and breeders continue to support the BVA/KC schemes and submit their dogs for testing.

DNA tests are normally applied to simple inherited conditions. Most inherited conditions use this type of inherence; only relatively few of those identified so far have a more complex mode of inheritance. Using these tests it is possible to determine if a particular dog is clear or affected by the disease, or whether it is a symptomless carrier that can nevertheless potentially pass the condition on to its offspring. A list of breed-specific official Kennel Club DNA testing schemes and dogs tested under these schemes can be found on the KC website.

DNA tests used in these schemes can accurately identify clear, carrier and affected dogs, and can be used by breeders to effectively eliminate undesirable disease genes in their stock. By publishing these results, on the UK Kennel Club website for instance, it also allows breeders to have a better understanding of which genes a dog may pass on to its offspring, giving them the information required to avoid producing affected puppies. Making informed decisions from health test results enables breeders to adapt their breeding programmes and reduce the risk of this disease appearing in future generations.

It is important to remember that every dog is most likely already a carrier for many autosomal recessive conditions. DNA tests are available for only a small number of the known mutations in dogs, but there are likely to be many more recessive mutations that we currently know nothing about. As well as taking into consideration health test results, the general health and performance of each parent, and the inbreeding coefficient of the potential puppies that could be produced, it is important that the temperament of the dogs and their conformation should be borne in mind when deciding on which dogs to breed. It is also extremely important to consider the welfare

EXPECTED RESULTS FROM MATING DNA TESTED DOGS			
Bitch status	**Stud dog status**		
	Clear	Carrier	Affected
Clear	All puppies in litter normal/clear	50 per cent of litter will be normal/clear, 50 per cent of litter will be carriers	All puppies in the litter will be carriers
Carrier	50 per cent of litter will be normal/clear, 50 per cent of litter will be carriers	25 per cent of litter will be normal/clear, 50 per cent of litter will be carriers, 25 per cent of litter will be affected	50 per cent of litter will be normal/clear, 50 per cent of litter will be affected
Affected	All puppies in the litter will be carriers	50 per cent of litter will be normal/clear, 50 per cent of litter will be affected	All puppies in litter affected

impact of any particular inherited condition; diseases with a high impact, having severe consequences causing significant pain, suffering and lasting harm, are best avoided whereas those with a low welfare impact might be better tolerated.

A simple chart illustrating the outcome of various mating strategies that can be applied when deciding on mating tested dogs is shown above.

It can be seen that even if a dog is a carrier it does not preclude its use for breeding, particularly within the numerically small breeds. As long as the gene is what's known as an 'autosomal recessive', mating carriers to 'clear' dogs will result in symptomless puppies, albeit they too will carry and pass on the gene to their progeny.

Health testing and the application of informed breeding strategies provide a means of controlling hereditary diseases and maintaining a healthier gene pool.

MATING THE BITCH

Traditionally dog breeders rely on a variety of signs associated with oestrus ('heat') to determine when to mate a bitch. These include mating at predetermined intervals, typically when she is ten to fourteen days after the first signs of heat, and/or observing or recording changes in the vulva and vagina. Unfortunately mating bitches at the wrong time using these methods still remains the most common cause of canine infertility because the ideal time to mate is just after she has ovulated (the time when eggs are first released from the bitch's ovaries) and this is sometimes earlier or later in her season.

The success in using these traditional methods can be attributed to the remarkable ability of dog sperm to survive in the female reproductive tract for up to seven days and for ova to be available for up to five days after ovulation. The fertile period in bitches can extend from five days prior to ovulation to five days following ovulation and it is possible for a mating at any time during this ten-day period to result in a pregnancy.

The point at which eggs are released from the ovaries into the fallopian tubes is known as ovulation and in order to optimize the chance of a successful pregnancy, it is necessary to determine the time of ovulation. If mating coincides more closely with the availability of fertile, mature eggs in the bitch's uterus it will not only optimize the chance of pregnancy but also the number of pups born of that mating.

Fortunately a greater understanding in our knowledge of the endocrine and physiological changes during the reproductive cycle in dogs has enabled the development of specific blood tests to help indicate the time of ovulation. Your vet will be able to collect the necessary blood samples, submit these for testing, provide information on how to interpret the results and consequently advise on when to mate your bitch. To

make best use of these tests, however, it is helpful if you have a little understanding of the endocrine changes occurring during oestrus and their influence on reproductive physiology in bitches.

The reproductive cycle of the bitch

Anoestrus is the period in which no external signs of ovarian activity are evident; the period when a bitch is neither in heat nor pregnant, nor, if not pregnant, undergoing some form of pseudopregnancy. Throughout anoestrus the reproductive tract is quiescent, the external genitalia, including the teats, appear their smallest size and levels of the hormone oestrogen remain relatively low. Immediately towards the end of anoestrus, oestrogen levels rise and this increase in circulating oestrogen induces the first signs of heat as the bitch enters pro-oestrus, the next phase of the cycle.

Pro-oestrus is evident as the characteristic progressive enlargement of the vulva and the appearance of a blood-tinged discharge accompanied by behavioural changes. The bitch becomes more and more attractive to male dogs, exhibits urine marking and, occasionally, a tendency to roam. Whilst the bitch may become more attractive to male dogs, she will refuse to allow them to mount, sometimes quite aggressively. During pro-oestrus, follicles start to develop in her ovaries under the stimulation of two hormones: follicular stimulating hormone (FSH) and luteinizing hormone (LH). These ovarian follicles also start to secrete oestrogen and as a result circulating levels continue to rise and the bitch passes into the next (receptive) phase that we know as oestrus.

Oestrus is defined by the behaviour of the bitch and is characterized by sexual attractiveness and the acceptance of male dogs, allowing them

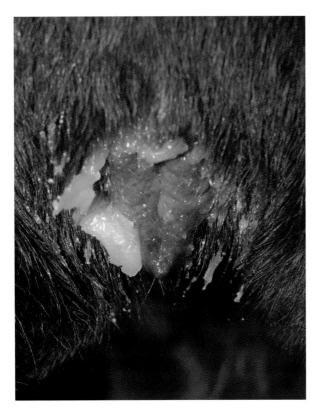

The characteristic appearance of the vulva of an in-season bitch, which swells considerably during oestrus. This bitch is ready to be mated and her vulva is smeared with Vaseline to provide lubrication and assist the stud dog in penetrating.

to mount and mate. Oestrogen levels are initially high but then decline, with a corresponding increase in the levels of another important hormone called progesterone. This coincidental decrease in oestrogen and rise in progesterone facilitates full expression of behavioural oestrus and the significant change in the ratio of these two hormones stimulates a dramatic rise in the level of LH immediately prior to ovulation.

These hormonal changes, particularly the pre-ovulatory LH surge, are highly predictive of ovulation; ovulations appear to occur synchronously about two days (thirty-six to fifty hours) after the LH peak. Whilst in most bitches ovulation occurs approximately twelve days after the beginning of pro-oestrus, it can occur as early as day five and in others as late as day twenty-five. Whilst a test for LH is not readily available, it is possible to test for progesterone and since an increasing level of progesterone in the blood is indicative of the imminent LH surge, by estimating the level of progesterone it is possible to predict the time of ovulation.

Progesterone testing therefore offers a distinct advantage when it comes to determining the best time to mate your bitch, particularly if she happens to ovulate either earlier or later than the expected norm. Simple qualitative or semi-qualitative progesterone test kits have become commercially available; by colloquial convention these are collectively referred to as 'the pre-mate test'. The kits are easy to use and the test requires no special expertise to perform. The result obtained is based on determining a simple colour change and the results are usually obtainable within thirty to forty-five minutes of collecting a blood sample, making it extremely convenient for use in general veterinary practice.

Unfortunately one pitfall of using the pre-mate test is that once the level of progesterone exceeds a certain concentration, which in the bitch persists for two months into the next phase of the cycle, it is possible to misinterpret the test result as 'mate immediately'. The test is only reliable if a pre-ovulatory sample has first been obtained, so ideally at least two samples are required: one prior to ovulation and a second at the time of or immediately following ovulation. If at the time of taking the first sample a 'mate immediately' result is obtained then other tests should also be performed to help confirm the result.

Quantitative laboratory blood test results give a much more accurate indication of progesterone concentration and are normally to be recommended. Typically the samples need to be sent to a commercial laboratory for testing, but the short delay in obtaining the result is usually unimportant because the bitch's ova need time to mature after ovulation before they can be successfully fertilized and mating need not be performed immediately.

Progesterone levels approximately double every day during this period. Once the level in the bloodstream reaches 15–24 nanomoles per litre (5–8 nanograms per millilitre) ovulation will occur and the bitch should be mated twenty-four to thirty-six hours later.

Normally it is recommended that the first sample should be taken seven days after the first sign of heat. The result thus obtained can determine when best to submit any further samples and since it is necessary to determine the rate at which progesterone levels rise prior to ovulation, it is not a good idea to rely on the result of a single sample unless that result indicates that the bitch is ready to be mated.

A further advantage of determining the time of ovulation is that it can be used to more accurately predict the date of whelping. Delivery of the first pup almost always occurs sixty-one to sixty-three days after ovulation.

Progesterone testing: interpreting the results

Depending on which laboratory is used to analyse the blood sample taken by your vet, the results will be expressed as either nmol/l (nanomoles per litre) or ng/ml (nanograms per millilitre). The following protocol expresses progesterone in nmol/l.

To convert these results to progesterone expressed as ng/ml MULTIPLY by 3.18 = progesterone in nmol/l; to convert nmol/l to ng/ml, DIVIDE by 3.18 = progesterone in ng/ml.

0–2 nmol/l Baseline concentrations; too early to estimate ovulation

3–6 nmol/l Minimum two days before ovulation is expected; however, result of 3–4 nmol/l may persist for a week or longer before increasing. Earliest estimated breeding four to six days later but could be longer (retest needed)

7–12 nmol/l Minimum one day before ovulation. Estimated window for breeding three to five days but could be longer (retest recommended)

13–18 nmol/l Ovulation impending or just occurred. Mate the bitch within the next two to four days

19–31 nmol/l Ovulation recently occurred. Mate the bitch within the next twenty-four hours to three days

32–64 nmol/l Ova have matured, optimal potential for fertility. Mate the bitch immediately and certainly within two days

65–90 nmol/l Mate the bitch immediately; however, ova have matured and ageing, decreased potential for fertility

Above 90 nmol/l Too late

The mating process

For most dogs, mating is a natural process. Occasionally, inexperienced dogs need a little help. The time of mating, the general health and condition of the dog(s) and environmental considerations are all important to the success of a natural breeding. With advances in techniques for veterinary assisted reproduction, however, breeders these days can choose to use alternative means to accomplish a breeding.

Traditionally dog breeders in the UK have relied solely on natural mating and this continues as the most popular means of achieving pregnancy in bitches. However, for health and welfare purposes, and also to diversify the gene pool, many dog breeders are now using artificial insemination to achieve pregnancy and these techniques will be described later, in Chapter 6.

So assuming you have selected a stud dog well in advance and the owner has agreed to the mat-ing, your bitch has come into season, and you have informed the stud dog owner, what next?

Firstly you to need to determine when your bitch will be ready for mating, either by recognizing signs to indicate that she is ready to accept the male and/or by using pre-mate blood tests to estimate the time of ovulation. Keep the stud owner informed so he or she can anticipate when their dog will be needed. Many stud dog owners will also work so bear this in mind when determining a time that will be suitable. If they live some distance away you may have to leave your bitch with the stud dog owner for a day or two to be mated. If this is the case, it needs to be organized well in advance.

It is customary to take the bitch to the stud dog. This is primarily because taking a male dog away from his home territory will tend to induce a sense of insecurity, his attention will wander and he will become preoccupied with scent marking and other distracted behaviours rather than remaining focussed on mating your bitch.

When going to have your bitch mated remember to take with you:

- The results of any health testing that you have carried out
- A copy of your bitch's pedigree
- A copy of the Kennel Club Litter Registration form, for the stud dog owner to sign
- The required stud fee.

The stud dog owner may require you to sign a contract, setting out the terms and conditions of their allowing the use of the dog at stud. If this is the case it is often helpful to see a copy of the contract in advance so you understand the requirement and will be happy to sign the contract.

Try to comply with the stud owner's preferences and suggestions, especially if it is an experienced breeder and particularly if this is your first opportunity to witness a mating and/or you have a 'maiden' bitch (one that has not been mated previously). Some stud dog owners insist that the bitch remains on a lead, especially if they have a particularly valuable stud dog. Others may want the bitch muzzled to reduce the risk of their dog

The actual process of canine copulation involves the male dog mounting the bitch from behind.

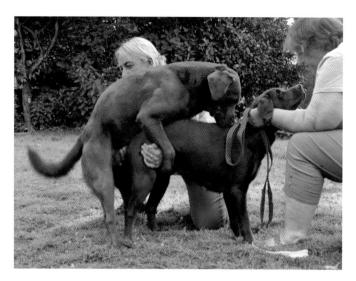

being bitten if there is any doubt that she is ready for mating.

The dogs should be afforded some privacy, ideally in a private enclosed area. Somewhere that offers a good footing so the dog doesn't slip whilst attempting to mount the bitch, and outside, weather permitting, where they will not be distracted.

Normally only two people are present and typically this will be the owners of the two respective dogs. Mating is a process that cannot be rushed. Dogs require time to become comfortable with each other; sometimes this will take several hours, even a day or so depending on their experience, disposition and the stage at which the bitch is in her oestrus cycle.

The female should show obvious signs of oestrus. She should flirt with the male dog, twitching her vulva and 'flagging' her tail by standing still, lowering her back and holding her tail closely to one side. The stud dog should appear to be very interested in the bitch, licking her vulva (to which she should show no objection) and repeatedly trying to mount her if she is ready and willing to allow him to do so. Talking to the dogs, using a soft, calm, soothing voice, will often help to make them feel more secure. If the female is unreceptive, she may sit or lie down, snap at the male dog, repeatedly retreat from him, or otherwise be uncooperative, particularly when he tries to mount.

At the point of penetration the canine penis is not fully erect and the stud dog is only able to enter the bitch's vagina because the penis includes a narrow bone, called the os penis. As the male penetrates, he will usually hold the female tighter and thrust deeply. At this stage the male's penis expands further and a structure, called the bulbus glandis, at the base of the penis, rapidly swells becoming trapped inside the female's vagina.

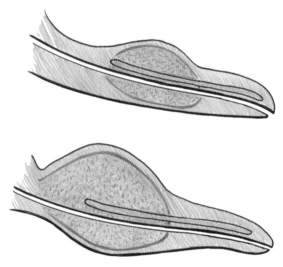

Diagrammatic representation of the canine penis to illustrate the relative size of the bulbus glandis in the normal (above) and erect penis (below).

Male dogs are the only animals that have a locking bulbus glandis or 'bulb', a spherical mass of erectile tissue at the base of the penis. During copulation, and only after the male's penis is fully inside the female's vagina, the bulbus glandis becomes engorged with blood. At the same time the female's vagina contracts and the dog's penis becomes locked inside the bitch; this is known as 'tying'.

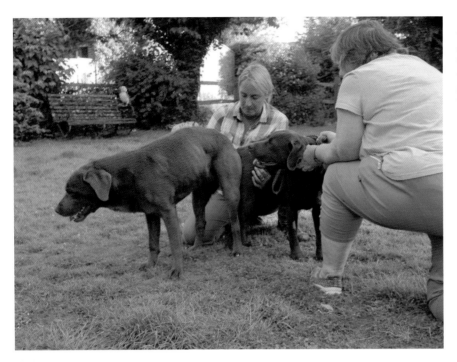

The copulatory tie. Once the stud dog's penis is fully engorged and locked within the female's vagina, he will typically turn and the two dogs will remain tied for fifteen to twenty minutes.

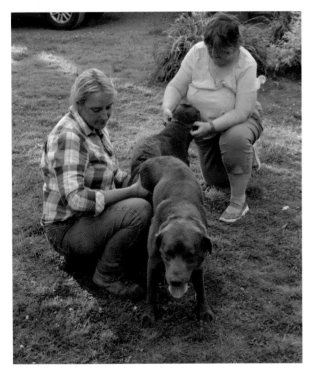

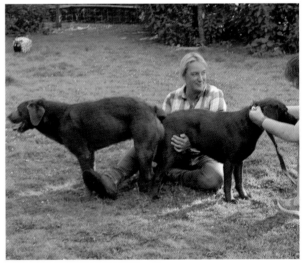

The mating process can be quite protracted and the stud dog handler and bitch owner might need to adopt a comfortable position whilst waiting for the dogs to finish tying.

Dogs remain tied during mating and will usually face away from each other during the process of insemination.

A dog's engorged penis is remarkably flexible and some dogs, as here, will turn to stand side-by-side whilst remaining tied.

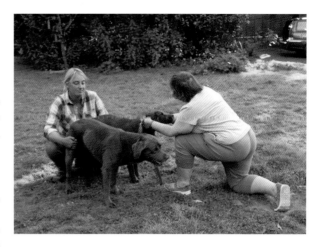

Once the copulatory tie is established, thrusting behaviour stops and the stud dog will usually lift a leg and swing it over the female's back whilst turning around. The two dogs then stand with their hind ends touching, the penis locked inside the vagina, while ejaculation occurs.

The precise purpose of the copulatory tie is unknown but no doubt originates in providing wild canines with some form of reproductive advantage. Canines are essentially pack animals and some believe the tie helps prevent competitive males from mating with the female. However, notwithstanding the influence of the pack hierarchy, they may subsequently do so and, if successful, could fertilize ova to produce a litter of mixed parentage. Certainly the total volume of a dog's seminal ejaculate is relatively large, and the tie would give the inseminating male's sperm a greater chance of fertilizing eggs and so passing on his genes.

Virgin bitches can become quite distressed during their first copulatory tie when they find they are unable to separate, and may try to pull away. It is helpful to attempt to calm such bitches using a soothing voice if they show anxiety once this stage is reached.

After some five to twenty minutes (but sometimes longer), the glans penis disengorges and contracts, allowing the dogs to separate and then, after mating, the stud dog usually cleans himself up by licking his penis and prepuce.

CONFIRMING PREGNANCY

There is no simple pregnancy test available for the bitch that an owner can conveniently use in the same way as there is for women. Pregnancy is normally confirmed by palpating the bitch about three to four weeks after she was mated and/or carrying out an ultrasound scan of her abdomen. This is best done by your vet, who will take this opportunity to check her over and provide you with any necessary advice on her care.

Manual palpation relies on being able to detect swellings in the uterine horns by palpating the bitch's abdomen. This is possible from three weeks through to five weeks of pregnancy. It is easiest in small- to moderate-size breeds that are not too prone to laying down abdominal fat. The developing pups are recognized as round, firm swellings rather like feeling a string of beads. As pregnancy progresses this becomes progressively more difficult as foetal fluid accumulates and it is often problematic if the litter is small.

Ultrasound examination is possible and foetal heartbeats can be identified quite early in pregnancy but as the exact timing of mating may be unknown, it is usually postponed until, or repeated at around three to four weeks of pregnancy.

Radiography is only reliable once the puppies' bones have developed and so it is only usual to X-ray bitches quite late in pregnancy, usually to confirm the number or position of the puppies prior to whelping.

Finally, there is a blood test for relaxin, a hormone unique to pregnancy since it is produced in the placenta (the point of attachment of the puppy, in its sac, to the wall of the uterus). The blood test can be used from around day twenty-five of pregnancy. A positive relaxin test reliably indicates that your bitch was definitely pregnant at the time the blood sample was taken. The test can be very helpful, especially in bitches that have previously 'failed to take', where, perhaps, they may have become pregnant initially but later resorbed the litter.

3 CARE OF THE BITCH DURING PREGNANCY

As we have seen, pregnancy in the bitch cannot be reliably detected until twenty-five to twenty-eight days, by which stage uterine swelling can usually be detected by ultrasound or palpation, or pregnancy confirmed by the measurement of serum relaxin concentration. Prior to about twenty-one days, the individual amniotic vesicles are small and difficult to palpate, especially in obese or tense dogs. After thirty-five days, increased amniotic fluid volume distends the vesicles and makes them confluent, obscuring their characteristic shape and turgidity.

Remember changes in early pregnancy related to progesterone are similar in both pregnant and non-pregnant bitches. All non-pregnant bitches go through a period of so-called pseudopregnancy after each season, although the related physical and physiological signs may differ from bitch to bitch and from one season to another in the same bitch.

It is important to understand that pregnancy, which is also referred to as gestation, only starts when the bitch's eggs are fertilized by the stud dog's sperm and not necessarily when the bitch is mated. A dog's sperm can survive for several days, sometimes up to a week, in the female reproductive tract giving the eggs time to be released from the ovaries and mature prior to fertilization. Consequently it is not essential to synchronize mating with the time of ovulation

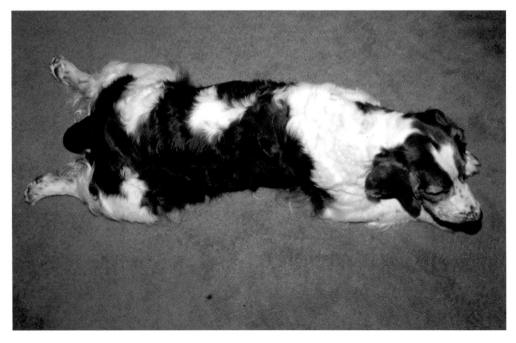

A bitch in the late stages of pregnancy. At this stage the gravid uterus occupies a significant proportion of the abdominal space.

(the release of eggs from the ovaries) for natural mating to be successful, although this does become more important when using artificial insemination (*see* Chapter 6).

Due to the variation in the time of ovulation between individual bitches (even between individual oestrus periods in the same bitch) whelping can be seen to occur at any time from fifty-seven to seventy-two days post-mating. More accurate measurements of gestational length in the dog are based on estimating the time of ovulation. Whelping occurs sixty-four to sixty-six days after the surge in circulating levels of leutinizing hormone, which precedes ovulation, so if blood sampling is used to determine the time of ovulation, whelping can be expected to occur some sixty-three days afterwards. There can, however, be some variation in gestation length depending on the breed and litter size, and a maiden bitch may sometimes have her puppies a few days early.

Implantation, the attachment of fertilized eggs to the wall of the uterus, usually occurs at around twelve to fourteen days post-ovulation and by three weeks post-ovulation the amnion and allantois, the foetal membranes, have formed. At this stage the embryo is approximately 5mm in length and the uterus itself slightly enlarged at the site of each placental attachment.

Although a pregnant bitch is regarded as being special she does not need to be spoilt, so following mating treat her essentially as normal albeit with due regard for her particular condition. The most vulnerable time for the fertilized eggs is prior to implantation and through the first three weeks of pregnancy. It is best to avoid exposing the bitch to any undue stress during this time and to any unnecessary risk of picking up infection.

It makes sense to take particular care with any bitch that could be pregnant to try to make sure that her mating has every possibility of resulting in the successful delivery of a healthy litter. We don't want to expose the bitch to anything that might be detrimental either to the establishment and development of her litter or to the health and subsequent welfare of her individual puppies. This is particularly important at the beginning and towards the end of pregnancy.

Once you know your bitch is pregnant you will need to take this into consideration, especially to determine how to feed and how much exercise to provide.

FEEDING THE PREGNANT BITCH

We all wish to do everything possible to ensure a pregnancy is successful and the resulting litter is healthy. It is understandable therefore that many people might be tempted to provide dietary supplements to their bitch, especially extra vitamins and minerals, to make sure she is in the best possible condition. Unfortunately this is incorrect. Excess vitamin and mineral levels can do a great deal of harm. There is no need to provide supplements, especially vitamins and minerals such as vitamin C and calcium, as any excess can cause harm.

Over-supplementing with vitamin C and calcium has been shown to cause skeletal effects in puppies and providing the bitch with extra, unnecessary, calcium prevents her being able to draw on her own reserves. This she will need to do when subsequently having to produce milk for her puppies and any interference with this physiological process will thus increase the risk of eclampsia (*see* Chapter 5).

Minimum dietary requirements have been established for most nutrients; however, the amounts will vary somewhat depending on the dog's stage of life (puppy, adolescent, adult, and senior) as well as whether pregnant or not. It is important to understand that these are the minimum requirements and as long as a bitch is already receiving a correct diet in adequate amounts, the increased food requirement of pregnancy and lactation will normally provide any additional nutrient requirements.

Based on these minimum requirements, guidelines have been developed as the general basis for the nutritional content of commercial pet foods. These of course are only guidelines and a particular dog may need more or less depending on its individual needs, circumstances and health status. As a further complication, in recent years nutritionists and veterinary researchers have identified that there are definite breed variations in metabolism and nutrient requirements. Breeds of dogs that were developed in specific locations may have adapted to specialized diets. Inbreeding and genetic differences between individuals can result in a further need for individualization of the dog's diet in order to optimize health.

When it comes to feeding, once you know your bitch is pregnant ensure she is fed high-quality food. Always feed a pregnant bitch the highest-quality food you can afford. The differences between a premium food and budget food aren't necessarily obvious on the label; they're found in the quality and source of the ingredients. Two dog foods, for example, may each contain a similar 27 per cent level of protein but can be vastly different when it comes to digestibility.

Avoid overfeeding through early pregnancy as this will simply encourage the bitch to lay down fat but once she is around six weeks pregnant, increase her feed intake incrementally by about 10 per cent per week so that by the time she is due to whelp she is consuming 50 per cent more than her normal amount.

You may find it helpful to utilize one of a variety of body condition scoring systems that have been devised for dogs to determine any adjustment required in your bitch's food intake or exercise requirement. Many are accessible online and a summarized example is outlined here.

BODY CONDITION SCORING

1 = Very thin
More than 20 per cent below ideal bodyweight.
Ribs, spine, hip bones and all body prominences easily seen (in short-haired dogs).
No discernible body fat can be felt beneath skin.
Obvious loss of muscle bulk.

2 = Thin
Between 10 and 20 per cent below ideal bodyweight.
Ribs easily felt and may be visible with no palpable fat. Spine visible. Hip bones less prominent.
Obvious waist and abdominal tuck.
Very little fat can be felt under the skin.

3 = Ideal
Ribs, spine and hip bones easily felt.
Visible waist and abdominal tuck.
Very little fat can be felt under the skin.

4 = Stout
General fleshy appearance.
Ribs, spine and hip bones difficult to feel.
Waist barely visible with a broad back, abdominal tuck may be absent.
Layer of fat on belly and at bottom of tail base.

5 = Obese
Ribs, spine and hip bones difficult to feel under a thick layer of fat.
Large fat deposits over chest, spine and tail base.
No waist can be seen and belly may droop significantly.
Heavy fat deposits on lower back and base of tail.

Types of feed

Complete feeds are the most popular choice for dog owners in the UK. Being 'complete', they contain all the nutrients required by a dog in the appropriate quantities to keep it fit and healthy. This means they can, and generally should, be fed alone. Proprietary brands often produce a special diet for pregnant and lactating bitches. Complete foods can be fed 'dry', when it is essential that you provide a readily accessible source of clean drinking water, or as a mash, normally mixed with hot water and allowed to cool before feeding. Feeding a dry food as a mash helps to prevent the stomach swelling up too much after the meal has been consumed as the dry feed starts to absorb gastric juices. This becomes increasingly important towards the end of pregnancy when the gravid uterus starts to take up a growing amount of space in the abdominal cavity.

Complementary foods are foods that do not contain the full range of essential nutrients or contain them in inappropriate proportions. For this reason other foods must be included in the diet. These other components can be home-prepared food, or mixer biscuits, a combination of both, or a complete food.

Many dog breeders seem to increasingly favour feeding frozen raw foods (see below) that mixers can effectively complement to provide a satisfactory balance of nutrients.

Raw feeding is regarded by many as the most natural way to feed a dog, and over the past few years has undergone something of a renaissance to become a very popular means of feeding dogs in the UK. It is especially useful for feeding to puppies after weaning when it can be conveniently mixed with a complementary mixer meal.

The term 'raw feeding' seems to be interpreted by some people, particularly those that criticize the practice, as equating to feeding with uncooked chicken carcasses. That is not what is intended. Here I refer to the feeding of uncooked food items that are otherwise suitable for consumption. Raw chicken carcasses are not recommended for feeding to dogs, especially

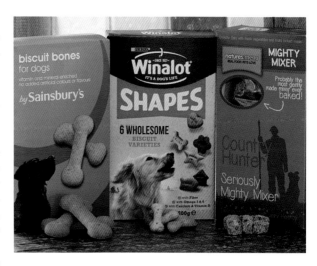

Mixer biscuits are cereal-based complementary foods that are sometimes flavoured with vegetables or herbs. They are nutritionally incomplete so need to be fed alongside a wet or raw food.

pregnant and lactating bitches and young puppies, because unless properly sourced and suitably processed, chicken meat can be a cause of bacterial food poisoning.

Many people prepare their own raw feed for their dogs, typically using frozen ingredients, but a number of companies have developed pre-prepared complete raw foods in the form of frozen blocks or nuggets, which provide all of the benefits of raw feeding with the convenience of a conventional dog food. There are both complete and complementary forms of raw foods and like wet foods, they inevitably contain a high proportion of water.

Whichever type of food you feed the bitch, offer her two or three smaller meals each day and if you feed a dry diet it is often wise to consider moistening the feed and offering it as a mash. In later pregnancy the gravid uterus can lead to displacement of the stomach with delayed and reduced gastric emptying; this can lead to the bitch requiring smaller, more frequent meals, especially as in the later stages of pregnancy her absolute requirements for carbohydrate and protein increase.

Some bitches show a tendency to go off their food two or three weeks after mating. This is quite natural and along with periodic vomiting may simply be a sign of early pregnancy similar to humans. Normal appetite will usually resume but if you are concerned, you might wish to consult with your veterinary surgeon. Avoid tempting the bitch to eat by offering treats and other tasty morsels. This will only tend to make her a 'picky' eater at a time when she should be consuming an adequate and balanced diet.

EXERCISING THE PREGNANT BITCH

Clearly the pregnant bitch needs to remain fit, healthy and in good bodily condition.

Don't underestimate the value of a good walk but do recognize that whilst jogging and running might be good exercise for us, dogs don't naturally engage in similar sustained exercise. A dog will typically engage in short bursts of activity, interspersed with intermittent stops. During these stops the dog will do such things as sniff around the immediate environment, defecate and urinate, rest and generally 'take in the scenery'.

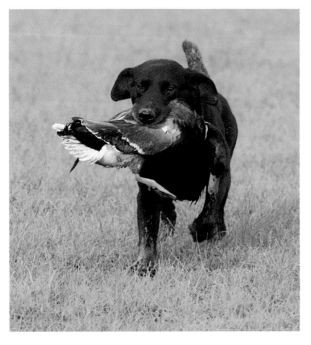

At least one good outing per day will help keep the bitch physically fit and otherwise help to relieve boredom. A walk should give her an opportunity to explore the wider world so that she experiences novel sights and smells.

Don't work or otherwise exercise a pregnant bitch until she has had ample time to digest a meal. This is especially important in the deeper-chested breeds and particularly towards the latter half of pregnancy when the enlarged uterus starts to compete for space in the abdomen.

In later pregnancy the gravid uterus can lead to cranial displacement of the diaphragm and decreased functional lung capacity.

WORKING AND SHOWING BITCHES IN WHELP

Regular moderate exercise and sufficient suitable feed will be important and in this respect there is no reason why, with care and consideration, a bitch cannot remain working during the early stages of pregnancy. Under normal circumstances pregnancy isn't generally confirmed until four weeks after mating and there is no evidence to suggest that non-strenuous working exercise during this period is likely to be detrimental. Of course with due deference to those with male dogs, do keep a mated bitch away from a shoot until the end of her heat period. Should the bitch go out of season early, however, it is usually a good sign that the mating has been successful. Don't allow her to become chilled and certainly ensure she doesn't become too hot, because this is known to cause deformities in puppies.

Once pregnancy is confirmed the precautionary principle must apply and great care should be taken not to submit the bitch to any form of strenuous exercise. If a few easy retrieves can be incorporated as part of a regular moderate

There seems to be no good reason not to work a bitch after mating and during the first few weeks of pregnancy. However, once pregnancy has been confirmed the precautionary principle should apply and strenuous exercise should cease.

daily exercise regime then it might be appropriate to continue a little longer, but certainly not beyond six weeks. Take care to avoid ground that is particularly challenging and where the going is heavy. If in doubt leave the bird for the pickers-up or for a colleague's dog to retrieve. Let the bitch determine the amount of exercise she requires; she will soon indicate when she is tiring, and of course offer her a small amount of water to drink at regular intervals.

There does not seem to be any evidence to support a ban on healthy bitches attending conformation shows in the early stages of pregnancy, and since pregnancy cannot be reliably confirmed until around four weeks any such ban would be impossible to enforce.

There would appear to be some evidence to suggest that pregnant bitches may undergo physiological stress if participating in strenuous physical activity (agility or flyball) and while it would be difficult to enforce a ban, owners should be reminded of their responsibilities under the Animal Welfare Act and advised not to compete.

In view of the potential risks of infection in mixing with large numbers of dogs and particularly of exposure to canine herpes virus (CHV), owners of pregnant bitches which attend shows, or come into contact with other dogs that attend shows, should be advised to contact their veterinary surgeon to discuss herpes virus vaccination.

Although there is no clear regulation regarding the transport of pregnant bitches, it may be appropriate advice that they are not transported to shows or other events from day forty-nine (seven weeks) after mating.

WORMING

Using modern worming preparations means it is safe to worm your bitch during pregnancy. Ask the advice of your veterinary surgeon and always use the dose and frequency he or she prescribes for the use of a particular product.

Worming during pregnancy is advised because products are now available that will eliminate encysted worm larvae in the bitch preventing their migration to infest developing puppies in her uterus during pregnancy as well as via the

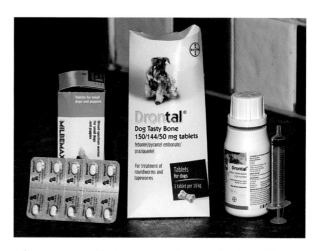

Always ensure that any worming product used is suitably licensed as being safe to use in pregnant bitches.

milk during lactation. Preventing puppies from becoming infested in this way will help ensure they do not suffer a heavy worm burden, that they will consequently be much healthier and that they will grow and develop better.

COAT CARE

The concept of 'grooming' might seem alien to many owners of gundogs and other working dogs because the term is more normally associated with dogs that require regular bathing, brushing and combing to keep them looking their best. What we are really considering here is maintaining good healthy skin and coat, the influence of pregnancy (and subsequent lactation) on a bitch's coat and any necessary trimming in preparation for whelping.

A dog's coat grows in three distinct cycles comprising an active growth phase, termed 'anagen', in which the hair reaches its genetically determined length, a transient 'catagen' phase and finally a resting phase termed 'telogen'. During pregnancy this cyclical growth is altered and all the hairs making up the coat enter the growth phase. As a consequence the bitch tends to grow a good coat whilst she is pregnant but after she has whelped a considerable amount of this coat will be shed.

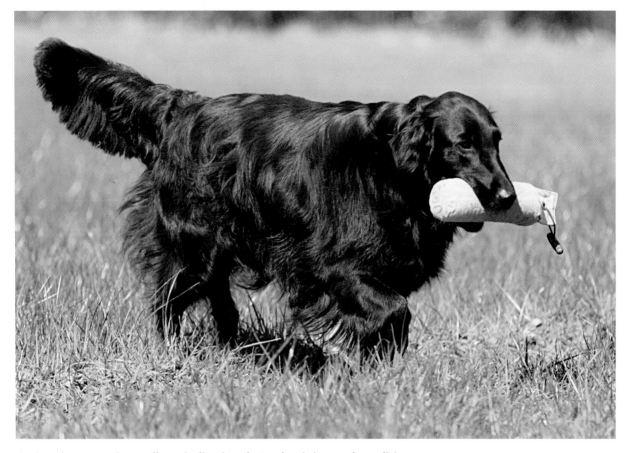

A nice glossy coat is usually an indication that a dog is in good condition.

Brushing (and combing as necessary) is probably the most important component of coat care, especially during pregnancy as this will remove dead hair, stimulate blood flow in the skin and help stimulate new hair growth. As a general rule, long-haired breeds should be brushed twice a week and bitches otherwise prone to moulting should be brushed approximately once a week. Remember the purpose of brushing is partly to remove superficial dirt and mud, dead coat and stimulate the skin.

Some dogs, gundogs especially, are quite content without a bath, particularly if they swim periodically. Do consider what they are swimming in of course, especially when they are pregnant. It is particularly important to avoid the chilling effect when a hot dog jumps into a pond

and remember that pond water isn't necessarily clean or fresh. Avoid bathing a pregnant bitch too often but if you have to bathe her, wherever possible use a mild shampoo or baby bath. Beware of using insecticidal shampoos because the active ingredient can be licked off or otherwise absorbed through the skin and potentially harm the developing puppies. Seek the advice of your veterinary surgeon.

Periodically run a comb through the coat and otherwise inspect for parasites such as fleas, lice and ticks. Use a flea comb to check for flea infestations and to search for loose ticks, especially in longer-haired dogs.

Just prior to whelping the coat should be trimmed in dogs that have 'feathering' – long hair on their ears, behind the legs, in front of the

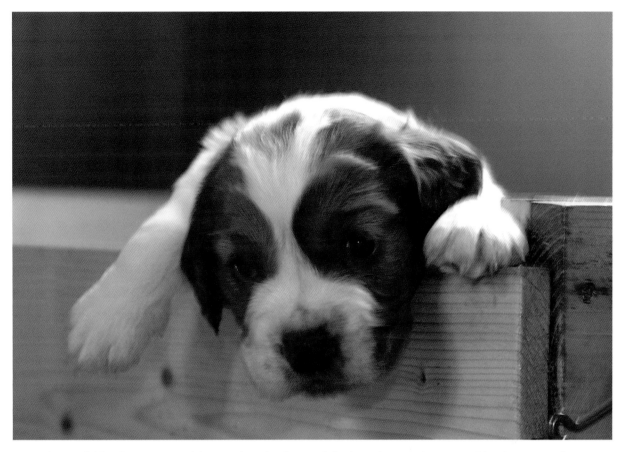

It can be useful having a removable panel at the front of the box that can be secured in place once the puppies have found their feet and become more active.

chest and under the chest and belly – especially the hair from around the vulva, behind the hind legs and from under the abdomen and around the teats.

PREPARING FOR WHELPING (WEEKS SEVEN TO NINE OF PREGNANCY)

Once the bitch is six to seven weeks pregnant, you should be making active preparations for whelping. By seven weeks the bitch's uterus will have enlarged to such a degree that adjacent foetuses are in contact and the individual swellings previously palpable in the abdomen are no longer apparent. By this stage there has been significant ossification of the vertebral bodies and some long bones in the foetus can be seen on

X-ray. The gravid uterus will be taking up more and more space in the abdomen and the bitch's body is otherwise adjusting to meeting the demands of her developing puppies. Her blood volume will increase, for instance, and this greater amount of diluted blood represents a mild anaemia. These are all normal adaptive changes but demonstrate how a pregnant bitch becomes more susceptible to stress and serves to emphasize how work or any other form of strenuous exercise should cease.

During this time acquire or make a suitable size whelping box. These are available to purchase and some are designed to be disposable once no longer required. A collapsible design can be stored for future use. Many breeders still prefer to use the traditional wooden whelping

CONSTRUCTING A TRADITIONAL WOODEN WHELPING BOX

The whelping box shown is made from pieces of timber 6in wide × $^3/_8$in thick, measures 36in wide × 30in deep, and is 12in high. The base is made of marine plywood, cut to size, and the corners are reinforced with strips of ½in square softwood. All joints are screwed and glued, then sealed with polyurethane varnish.

To construct this box you will need:

One piece 36in × 30in × ½in marine plywood
Five softwood planks, each approximately 6ft long × 6in wide × $^3/_8$in thick
Two softwood planks, each approximately 6ft long × 4in wide × $^3/_8$in thick
Two softwood strips approximately 6ft long × ½in square
Two softwood strips approximately 6ft long × ½in × $^3/_8$in
Two brass hooks and eyes
Approximately 48 brass wood screws
Wood glue and polyurethane varnish
Saw, drill and bit, screwdriver, sandpaper and a paint brush

1. Start by cutting out the base. Use good-quality marine plywood. Glue and screw pieces of ½in square strip around the edges as seen in the photograph; this creates an insulating air gap under the floor of the box. Use brass screws throughout, which won't rust.

2. Cut and assemble pieces of timber to form the sides and back with a single piece to form the front as shown in Figure 1. Use a ½in square strip for the corner supports to which you can screw and glue the panels. Further strips are attached to the inside of the back and sides, level with the top of the front panel; these will support the ledge inside the box as shown in Figure 2.

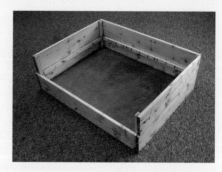

Fig. 1 The basic box with strips attached to the inside of the back and sides to support the removable ledge.

3. Cut suitable lengths of 4in × $^3/_8$in timber to form the side and back ledges; a piece of 6in × $^3/_8$in timber is used for the front ledge. Assemble the ledge on a flat surface. Glue together, and screw and glue two ½in square strips under each side panel and to the front and back panels to provide rigidity. Set aside to dry thoroughly.

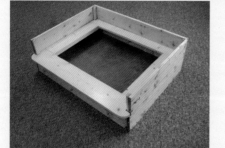

Fig. 2 The whelping box with the ledge in situ that will help prevent the bitch from lying on her puppies.

4. When the glue is dry, assemble the ledge inside the box, cutting out squares in appropriate positions so that the ledge slides neatly down past the ½in square strips in the corners of the whelping box.

5. Complete the assembly by making the removable front panel from 6in × ³/₈in timber, cut to size – this will help your pregnant bitch enter the box safely. This panel can be secured to the box using hooks attached to each side and eyes screwed into each end of the front panel.

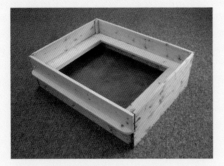

Fig. 3 A removable front panel will facilitate the bitch entering and exiting the box, especially when heavily lactating.

6. Finally, give all the surfaces several coats of suitable clear polyurethane varnish. Apply sufficient coats to seal all the joints, particularly those on the inside of the box.

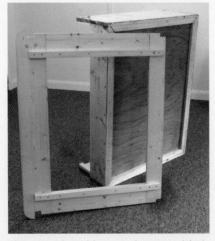

Fig. 4 The completed box and removable ledge should be given several coats of polyurethane varnish. This helps to seal the wood and all the joints and makes it easier to clean and disinfect the box whilst in use and prior to accommodating any subsequent litters.

box, which is warmer for the puppies compared to newer, more clinically clean, materials. The whelping box should be around 12in high and have a ledge or rails around the inside walls that enable puppies to avoid being inadvertently squashed if the bitch chooses to lie up against the side of the box. Try to make it in such a way that there is an insulating air gap between the base of the box and the underlying floor. It is useful if the front of the box, above the rail, can be removed to allow the lactating bitch to get in and out comfortably.

If you decide to make your own box, make sure it is large enough for the bitch to stretch out. To determine a suitable length, the space between ledges or rails should be at least the length of the bitch from neck to rump; some bitches like to lie with their heads resting on a ledge. To decide on width, allow space for the bitch to lie with her back against the ledge or rail and extend her legs so they just touch the opposite side of the box.

If you construct the box out of wood, it should be varnished or painted to make it easy to clean and disinfect. Always use non-toxic varnish or paint, for example the type that would be suitable for children's toys.

Instructions for making a typical traditional wooden whelping box, suitable to whelp the average medium-size breed of dog, are outlined and illustrated in the box adjacent.

NESTING BEHAVIOUR

One of the consequences of pregnancy is the bitch's natural urge to create a cave-like structure in which to whelp. This is not to be confused with the so-called 'nesting' behaviour, in which the bitch attempts to tear up bedding prior to whelping and which is more likely to be a sign of mild to moderate discomfort as her uterus starts to contract in preparation for giving birth.

Individual bitches will vary in the extent to which they exhibit this behaviour. It is probably better not to suppress your bitch's natural instinct to dig but you do need to monitor the situation carefully.

You certainly don't want a situation where the bitch can get out of reach at the back of an extensive excavation so you are unable to retrieve her in the later stages of pregnancy, prior to parturition. Also care needs to be taken in lighter soils and in sandy ground to ensure she doesn't become trapped if the soil in her tunnel were to collapse. Terriers and other breeds that are accustomed to hunting rabbits need to be prevented from entering burrows when pregnant, since their increased girth might mean they are able to enter but unable to turn around and get out again.

MEDICATION

Except for using suitably approved worming products prescribed by your veterinary surgeon, it is generally advisable to avoid treating pregnant bitches with any form of medication unless absolutely necessary. Any medical treatment should only be that prescribed by your veterinary surgeon, who will be able to advise on the use of products that are specifically licensed as suitable for use in pregnant bitches.

DISEASE RISKS ASSOCIATED WITH PREGNANCY

A number of diseases can develop as a result of pregnancy. These principally include pregnancy toxaemia, eclampsia, hypertension and diabetes mellitus. Each of these conditions is more likely to be seen in the later stages of pregnancy or during lactation and are described in Chapter 5.

Concurrent disease can also affect the pregnancy and result in resorption of the developing foetus, abortion or foetal retention at parturition and subsequent mummification of the retained foetus.

Resorption can be complete, when the whole litter is affected and pregnancy effectively terminates, or partial where just one or two conceptuses are resorbed and pregnancy continues. The incidence of resorption is unknown although one study involving stray dogs indicated that 40 per cent of bitches showed evidence of resorption and that pregnancy continued in over 80 per cent. Whilst incidence rates are more likely to be very much lower in well-cared-for domestic dogs, one

study indicated that resorption can occur in 5–11 per cent of pregnancies and that foetal resorption is recognized as one of the causes of small litter size. The causes of resorption can include infection, trauma, foetal defects and maternal factors including ill health, the administration of certain drugs and the ingestion of toxins.

Canine herpes virus (CHV) is thought to be the most common cause of viral abortion in bitches and can cause neo-natal death in puppies within the first three days of life. The exposure of unprotected bitches to CHV during the last three weeks of pregnancy can result in the death of foetuses in utero or the loss of puppies for up to three weeks after parturition. Infection of normal, otherwise healthy adult dogs is probably asymptomatic and the animals remain as healthy carriers that only shed the virus periodically when either stressed or in heat. A significant proportion of the UK dog population therefore is probably immune under natural conditions. Transmission of infection occurs through direct contact with genital or oronasal secretions of infected dogs and the subsequent effect of infection will then depend on the stage of pregnancy at which infection occurs. Bitches in mid-gestation will probably abort or give birth to stillborn puppies without necessarily showing any other signs of infection. Some puppies may be born apparently healthy but then become ill and die due to infection within a few days of birth.

Other infections known to cause abortion and neo-natal death in dogs include canine parvovirus-1, canine distemper virus (CDV), and canine adenovirus-1 (CAV1). The two most common causes of bacterial abortion and neo-natal death in dogs are *Brucella canis* and *Streptococcal* infection. Infection with other bacterial organisms such as *Escherichia coli*, *Campylobacter* spp., *Leptospira* spp. and *Salmonella* spp. can also occur sporadically.

Physiological changes
During her pregnancy a bitch undergoes a variety of physiological changes that can adversely influence her health. Firstly, during gestation she is under the influence of the hormone progester-

one and this increased progesterone concentration has effects on glucose metabolism. This can lead to insulin resistance, gluconeogenesis and in some cases hypoglycaemia (low levels of circulating blood glucose) in late pregnancy, thereby putting the bitch at risk of developing canine gestational diabetes.

Secondly, a bitch's total circulating blood volume increases during her pregnancy and this gives rise to haemodilution, whereby normal constituents in the blood tend to become somewhat more diluted in the greater circulating volume. This in turn leads to a mild anaemia.

Canine gestational diabetes

A bitch suffering from canine gestational diabetes will develop high levels of blood sugar, which we refer to as hyperglycaemia. As a direct consequence sugar is present in her urine, a condition called glucosuria, which will result in excessive urination. The bitch will be extremely thirsty and to compensate will require a lot more water than she would normally drink; this, in turn, will cause her to pass more urine, more frequently. She will lack energy and show signs of weight loss even though she has an increased appetite. These symptoms will gradually become worse as the disease progresses. Early detection of the signs of gestational diabetes is vitally important to enable successful treatment of the bitch. Early detection, coupled with prompt medical treatment, will help ensure that the long-term prognosis for the bitch will normally be good, and the condition may well resolve once the bitch has given birth to her litter of puppies. It is likely to recur, however, if she has another pregnancy.

Pregnancy toxaemia

Hypoglycaemia of pregnancy or pregnancy toxaemia is a serious metabolic disease that occurs in undernourished pregnant bitches during the later stages of gestation. It is seen most commonly in thin, poorly conditioned bitches, especially those carrying very large litters. It is relatively uncommon.

A bitch must be fed an adequate diet, especially through the later stages of pregnancy. Any tendency to go off her food in the last twenty days of pregnancy must be quickly corrected because the puppies will double in weight during the last two weeks of gestation.

These bitches have inadequate fat reserves, muscle mass and are fed low carbohydrate diets. The disease occurs late in pregnancy when the developing litter is rapidly growing and the embryos are requiring higher levels of protein and fat than these bitches are able to supply. Since the diet is insufficient to provide all her energy requirements, the bitch will naturally try to break down her own protein and fat stores in order to maintain the pregnancy.

A by-product of excess protein and fat breakdown is high levels of ketones. These ketones are excreted in urine and exhaled through the lungs. If the situation is not corrected the bitch will become toxic due to the ketone levels in her bloodstream.

A bitch with pregnancy toxaemia will become lethargic and go off her food. Some people can smell the ketones on the dog's breath. A vet will use a urine dipstick test and if this reveals ketones, that confirms a diagnosis of pregnancy toxaemia.

In mild cases, early intervention and feeding a high-fat, high-protein supplement will correct the deficit. If pregnancy toxaemia becomes established, the goal is to get the bitch to term and to closely supervise whelping; a high percentage of ketotic bitches will lack sufficient energy to whelp the whole litter and the last few puppies may be born by caesarean. In severe cases, the bitch may have to be hand-fed to term when some litter losses are not uncommon. In extreme cases pregnancy may have to be terminated in order to save the bitch's life.

4 WHELPING AND THE CARE OF NEO-NATAL PUPPIES

PREPARING FOR WHELPING

About two weeks before the expected date of whelping, set up the box that you will have previously constructed or purchased, in the room selected as suitable for the bitch to give birth and care for her pups immediately afterwards. You are going to be spending some time in this room, so now is the time to clear yourself some space and make the area as comfortable as possible for both you and your bitch.

When deciding on which room to use, remember that the bitch is going to need access to your garden or somewhere similar to relieve herself from time to time and to return to continue looking after her litter. Ideally the area might have immediate access but otherwise just consider the route she has to take and how easy it will be for her to go outside and return.

Position the box where there is sufficient room to work and enough light for you to see what is happening and to check on the bitch and her puppies once they are born. The area needs to be free from draughts especially in winter, warm but not too hot. Similarly you may have to choose somewhere that you are able to keep reasonably cool in the summer. You are aiming to achieve a temperature within the whelping box of around 27–30°C (80–86°F).

The whelping area should be situated somewhere where it is quiet, warm with no draughts, with ample light and sufficient room for you and your bitch. Here, in the corner of a study, everything required is placed close at hand and an infrared light has been installed above the whelping box to provide supplemental heating for the puppies.

There needs to be room for the box and all the necessary ancillary equipment. Some people like to provide an infrared lamp as local heating for the puppies, although it is more effective to provide a heat source on which the puppies can lie, for example an electrical heat pad in one corner of the whelping box. Decide how you are going to position the heat lamp. You are going to need a convenient power socket and will want to be able to adjust the height of the bulb above the whelping box that will, in turn, determine how hot the area is beneath the lamp. It is often convenient to hang the lamp from a hook in the ceiling above the whelping box; alternatively you may be able to use an adjustable lamp stand as shown in the accompanying photograph.

You are going to require three to four pieces of suitable bedding, just large enough to fit in the bottom of the whelping box. Fleecy polyester bedding has become readily available and is ideal for the purpose. Originally marketed under the brand name 'Vetbed', this type of bedding is warm and fluffy for the bitch and puppies to lie on, and provides a non-slip surface, both for the bitch during parturition and for the puppies once they are up on their feet and starting to walk around. It tolerates frequent washing on a hot wash cycle in the washing machine and will last for a considerable length of time, so it is quite economical to use. Importantly it offers a semi-permeable membrane through which urine will pass so the surface remains dry. You will need at least three separate pieces because at any point in time you might have one piece in use within your whelping box, another in the wash, and a third piece drying. If you have a fourth piece then it is reassuring to know there is always some clean bedding available, ready for immediate use.

Lay out all that will be required so that everything is ready and to hand, should the bitch start whelping unexpectedly. Hopefully she will give you plenty of notice (*see below*) but occasionally a bitch will show little or no preparatory signs and suddenly start to whelp a puppy. In such circumstances you don't want to be rushing around looking for old towels to dry the puppy or something suitable to tie off the umbilical cord. All these things, and more, need to be assembled well in advance so they are available and ready for use at a moment's notice.

The following is a list of some ancillary items that you might wish to have available:

- Old newspapers, useful for lining the whelping box, placed under the bedding to absorb urine and so on
- Disposable surgical gloves (available from your vet)
- A nailbrush, soap and towels – so you can wash and dry your hands if you have to internally examine the bitch
- Old towels for drying the puppies
- A rectal/clinical thermometer
- Glucose and water for the bitch to drink (dissolve one tablespoonful of glucose in each pint of drinking water)
- Surgical scissors and artery forceps (or similar) to cut and clamp the umbilical cords
- Paper kitchen towel
- Plastic sacks in which to subsequently dispose of soiled materials
- Bottle feeder(s), bitch's milk replacer, sterilizing solution, bottle brushes and so on
- Scales to weigh puppies, notebook and pencil/pen
- A torch – in case the bitch needs to go outside at night
- Telephone hot number of your veterinary surgery
- Box with water bottle wrapped in towelling – in case you have to separate the puppies from the bitch, for example to take them with her to the vet.

THE PROCESS OF WHELPING

Towards the end of pregnancy the uterus becomes more and more crowded with developing pups and once the cervix dilates, the presence of the first puppy in the birth canal initiates the active, expulsive process of whelping.

Whelping is often conveniently described as taking place in three phases, but in fact there is a further preparatory phase. During this preparatory phase, the levels of the hormone progesterone which have been circulating in the bloodstream to maintain pregnancy and prevent the uterus from contracting down during the growth of the developing foetuses drop and circulating levels of the hormone oestrogen correspondingly start to rise and take over. At this point in time the production of another hormone, prostaglandin, is stimulated and whelping is initiated.

We believe that these hormonal changes are triggered by the rising cortisol levels produced by the developing foetuses, which are becoming more and more crowded in the uterus. While this is happening the bitch's body temperature will drop. This rapid and significant fall in body temperature is extremely helpful when it comes to pinpointing the start of whelping. To do this, record the bitch's rectal temperature two or three times daily, starting about four to five days prior to the expected date of whelping. A dog's normal body temperature is 38.6°C (101.5°F), however towards the end of a bitch's pregnancy it will tend to be a little lower than usual. Consequently when recording rectal temperature for the purpose of finding out when your bitch is whelping, work on the basis that her rectal temperature during this final week of pregnancy will likely be around 37.7°C (100°F) rather than the normal 38.6°C (101.5°F). You should then be able to detect a distinctive and significant further drop in temperature when it will rapidly fall to 37.2°C (99°F) or as low as 36.1°C (97°F), indicating that the bitch should whelp within the next twenty-four hours.

The time taken to give birth to a litter can be extremely variable. A fit, healthy young bitch can give birth in less than an hour; in others it can be very much more protracted with long intervals, sometimes several hours, between pups. Most working dogs will typically whelp over a period of two to six hours but there are no hard and fast rules.

THE FIRST STAGE OF WHELPING

During the first phase of whelping the bitch will become restless, start panting and usually refuse food for eighteen to twenty-four hours, and sometimes water, and may vomit. She may tear up her bedding, a sign of internal discomfort,

albeit traditionally described as 'nest-building'. Some people advocate providing the bitch with a pile of old newspapers precisely for this purpose but unfortunately many bitches will want to choose their own 'nesting' area and completely ignore your newspaper. Do watch the bitch whenever she is let out in the garden. As previously described, many bitches will choose to nest-build by digging under some convenient structure like your garden shed or by tunnelling into a bank. These excavated nesting holes can often become quite large and if you happen to be a keen gardener, you won't necessarily welcome the result of your bitch's instinctive nest-building behaviour.

Bitches vary in their behaviour through this first stage, which typically lasts as long as twelve to forty-eight hours but in some dogs can be remarkably brief. Individual bitches can also vary between different whelpings.

You may have noticed a slight mucoid discharge from the vulva during pregnancy. If this has been the case then just prior to whelping you might notice that this discharge increases and appears as 'strings' of mucous hanging from her vulva, indicating that the mucoid plug, previously sealing the cervix, has dissolved.

DYSTOCIA AND UTERINE INERTIA

Occasionally a bitch may go through the preparatory and first stages of whelping and then fail to whelp a puppy. A lengthy delay can result in the death of a puppy particularly if the placenta, the attachment of the puppy in its amniotic sac to the wall of the uterus, becomes detached, interrupting the supply of bitch's blood to the puppy. Failure of the uterus and cervix to contract and expand normally and/or to expel a foetus is called dystocia.

Remember it is the foetus, not the dam, that initiates the start of whelping. In bitches carrying an exceedingly small litter and especially those with just a single puppy, there may be insufficient stimulus to initiate whelping. Consequently the bitch fails to enter the second, expulsive stage and a caesarean section will be required to assure the birth of viable puppies.

Alternatively bitches with obviously large litters and displaying all the other signs of imminent whelping may be reluctant to start at all. This is usually due to primary uterine inertia. In this instance the uterine muscles fail to contract properly, either due to poor muscle tone, obesity, or general lack of fitness in the bitch. It can also occur if the uterus becomes over-stretched and thus unable to contract properly because it has expanded to its full capacity/capability in order to accommodate a large number of puppies. Primary uterine inertia can also be familial, due to hereditary factors and occurring within certain families and among dogs of particular breeds.

Secondary uterine inertia on the other hand is the term used for the cessation of uterine contractions and a failure to expel further foetuses following the birth of one or more puppies. The cause is often due to the uterine muscle becoming fatigued, especially during the birth of a large litter. In such circumstances a veterinary surgeon will usually administer oxytocin, a hormone normally produced by the pituitary gland that induces uterine contractions. An injection of oxytocin will therefore cause the uterus to contract almost immediately and thus expel any remaining foetuses. Occasionally the injection will have to be repeated. If there is no response to oxytocin then the veterinary surgeon will normally recommend carrying out a caesarean.

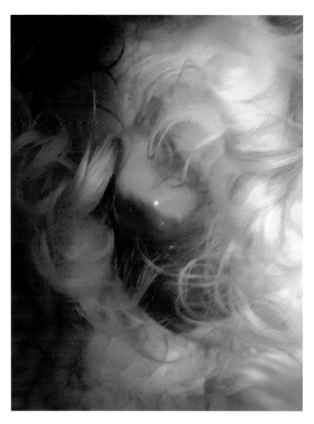

A good sign that a puppy is about to be born is the appearance of a glistening, fluid-filled sac at the vulva and part of the puppy, typically a nose as in this photograph, will be visible within the sac. (Photo: Wendy Buckwell)

THE SECOND STAGE OF WHELPING

During the first stage of whelping, the cervix, situated between the uterus and the vagina, will have opened to allow puppies to pass into the vagina during birth. Unless the cervix is dilated at this stage, a birth by natural means cannot occur. Unfortunately in dogs, unlike in many other species including women, there is no way of manually checking if the cervix is open because it is located high up, just inside the rim of the pelvis; too far forward to be reached with a finger.

As the bitch enters this second stage she stops panting and becomes quieter. You should see stronger abdominal contractions and that she is arching her back and pressing down with her rear end. Once she starts bearing down and actively straining, make a note of the time because there could be complications if this process goes on for too long without further progress. If a puppy has not been born within half an hour, take her out in the garden and see if walking around will help to 'stir things up'. If there is still no progress then phone your vet for advice, explaining for how long she has been straining.

The first noticeable sign of an impending birth will be the appearance of a dark fluid-filled bag at the vulva. This is the amniotic sac; what is often referred to as the 'water bag'. This membranous sac has surrounded the foetus during pregnancy and now serves to help lubricate its passage through the birth canal. The bag may appear and

47

then retract a couple of times, so don't be concerned if this should happen. Eventually the bag bursts, sometimes higher up the vagina, when there will be a gush of fluid and the first pup should be born soon afterwards. The bitch may stand, crouch (and bear down), or lie down for the actual birth.

Pups 'dive' out of the birth canal, feet first, and can come out forwards (head first) or backwards with no problem. When the head or rear end is presented and no legs are obvious, problems can arise and in such circumstances manual assistance may be necessary to correct the presentation.

If there appears to be no expulsive progress once a puppy has appeared at the vulva, you may have to assist your bitch by applying gentle traction on the puppy. To do this, first thoroughly wash your hands or wear disposable surgical gloves because you do not want to introduce alien infection into the reproductive tract. With the back of your hand upwards, take the puppy between your first and second fingers, and as the bitch strains pull very gently downwards. It is important that you don't try to pull the puppy straight out, directly towards you. As you can see from the accompanying diagram, the angle of the birth canal is downwards from the pelvis, not straight out like the rectum, and it is important to pull gently in the direction taken by the puppy during the natural birth process.

Ease the puppy gently out of the vulva, if necessary with the aid of some lubricating jelly. Sometimes this is necessary with the first puppy presented but once this pup has passed through the pelvis, it will effectively enlarge the passage for the remainder of the litter.

It may be a little more difficult if this first puppy is coming out hind feet first as the widest part of the

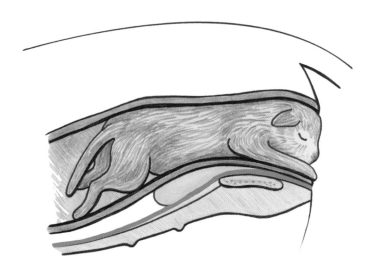

Normal presentation. The puppy presented head first with the forelimbs extended, ready to 'dive' out of the birth canal.

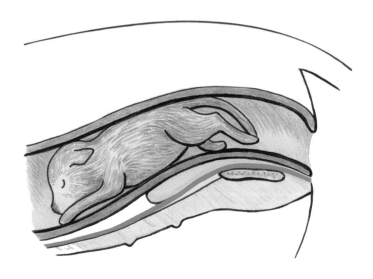

Normal presentation with the puppy presented backwards. Note the hind limbs are extended, enabling the puppy to slip relatively easily through the birth canal.

Schematic diagram of a cross-section of the bitch's pelvis, showing the relative position of the reproductive organs. Note how entry and exit to/from the birth canal is angled downwards; this has to be taken into account whenever assisting a whelping by helping a puppy pass out through the birth canal.

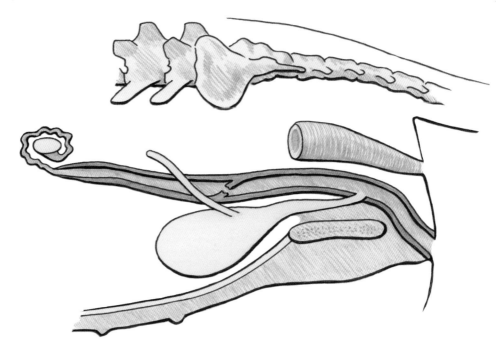

A breech presentation. The puppy is presented tail/rump first, with the hind limbs forwards. To correct the problem the puppy must be pushed back into the uterus and the hind limbs drawn backwards.

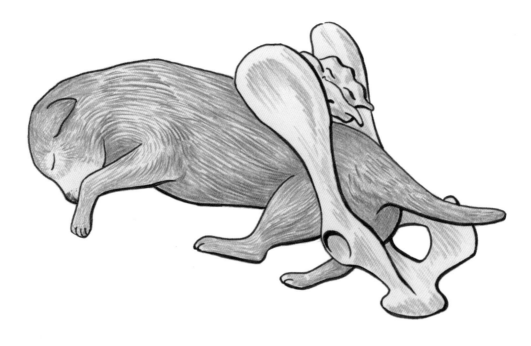

puppy, in this case the rump, is not leading the way. It is also more difficult because in a posterior presentation the puppy is passing out in the opposite direction to the natural lie of its fur. This presentation, with the puppy coming out hind feet first, is not a breech presentation as many people believe – a breech presentation is where the puppy is presented rump first with the hind legs tucked under the body, back inside the vulva. This is illustrated on the previous page and represents a much more difficult presentation to manually correct.

Approximately half of all puppies born will be presented hind feet first and unless it happens to the first one, or a particularly large puppy, this presentation will normally cause few problems.

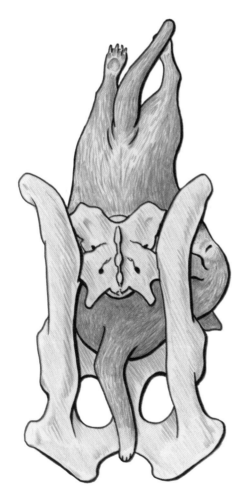

A puppy presented with its head deflected to one side will be unable to enter the birth canal and will require manual manipulation in order to correct the presentation before whelping can continue normally.

If the puppy is presented with its head deflected to one side or if one leg is pointing backwards, you may have to straighten up the puppy first in order for its birth to proceed smoothly. With a little lubricating jelly on your finger you should be able to ease the necessary part of the puppy back into the required presenting position. Don't be afraid to push the puppy back into the uterus a little at first, as this will provide more room for you to correct the position of whichever part of the body is impeding the puppy's progress.

Keep calm and try to imagine the normal anatomical presentation that you are attempting to restore. Don't be tempted to pull too strongly on an exposed limb or head; brute force won't help and simply risks causing an injury. A gentle pull timed to coincide with a bitch's contraction should be all that is required. You will find that digital pressure on the rim of the pelvis will stimulate the bitch to push and you might use this reflex, as necessary, to help you expel the puppy when you have your finger inside the birth canal.

With a puppy this close to being born, direct veterinary assistance is likely to be of little use because it is likely to be dead by the time your vet arrives. A call to the surgery, however, explaining the situation you are presented with may be useful if, from your description, the vet is able to understand the situation and help by talking you through the ways and means of correcting the presentation.

Once born, the priority is to get the puppy out of the amniotic sac so that it can breath. The bitch will normally tear the sac with her front (incisor) teeth, chew off the umbilical cord using the molar/premolar teeth at the side of her mouth and consume the foetal membranes, including the placenta if it has been expelled along with the puppy. The bitch will then set about resuscitating her puppy and stimulating it to breathe, turning it over and pulling on the umbilical cord. Don't be

Another abnormal presentation. In this case the puppy's head is deflected downwards and the top of the cranium is presented at the pelvic brim. The puppy will need to be pushed back into the uterus and the nose raised so that it can enter the pelvis and allow whelping to resume.

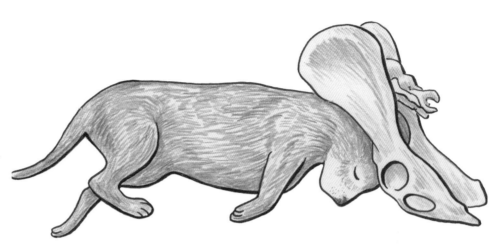

too concerned if she seems a little rough with her puppy at this stage. This is simply nature's way of encouraging the puppy to respond vigorously and to start breathing normally.

Most bitches will give birth unassisted with no trouble at all but many breeders prefer to 'whelp' their bitches, delivering and reviving each puppy by removing the placental attachments and foetal membranes, vigorously drying the pup to initiate respiration, and ensuring that each puppy suckles and thereby receives its vital colostrum – the first milk.

Do not be tempted to rush in, however; if possible let the bitch exhibit natural maternal behaviour as this will assist the bonding process, help her see the litter as being her own, assist the let-down of milk and generally help reinforce her natural maternal instinct throughout the period of lactation.

If the bitch should neglect the puppy, and some bitches with the first litter may be a little confused with all that is going on at first, then you will have to intervene. Tear the foetal membranes and hold the puppy upside down to drain fluid from its lungs. Then rub and dry the puppy vigorously with a towel to stimulate breathing. Clean the mouth and nostrils to clear the airway and finally attend to the umbilical cord.

Should the puppy fail to breathe, hold its head between your first two fingers and the puppy in

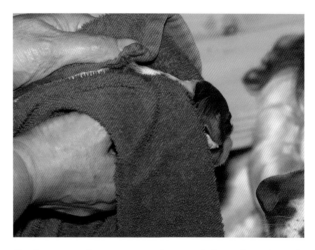

Drying a newborn puppy vigorously in a clean towel will help to stimulate breathing.

the palm of your hand. Swing the puppy, upside down, vigorously by your side. This will both clear the airway and gravitational force on the downswing should stimulate a reflex movement of the chest, encouraging the puppy to give its first vital gasp.

Once you are happy that the puppy is fully revived and breathing normally (unassisted), you can tie off the cord. To do this, first 'milk' blood back towards the puppy's tummy and clamp the

51

cord with forceps. Tear the cord with your fingers or cut the cord with scissors as far away from the puppy as possible. A little later you can remove the clamp and, using cotton thread, tie a ligature where the clamp has crushed the puppy's cord.

THE INTERVAL BETWEEN BIRTHS

Probably one of the most worrying aspects of whelping a bitch, particularly for less experienced breeders, is knowing how long it is safe to leave her between the birth of successive puppies

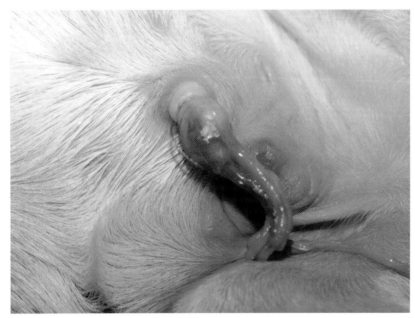

The umbilical cord of a newborn puppy which has been tied off with cotton thread.

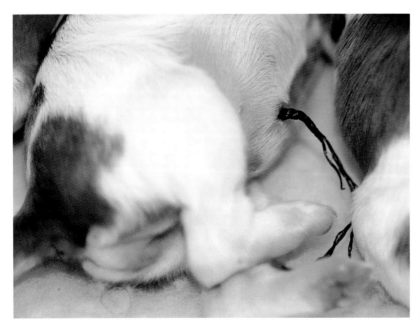

Once tied off and deprived of a blood supply, what remains of the umbilical cord will dry up and wither over the next few days and eventually fall off naturally.

before seeking veterinary assistance. The interval between the birth of normal live puppies can vary but you might reasonably expect to leave about two and a half to three hours between puppies before becoming unduly alarmed and calling the surgery.

You should have alerted the veterinary practice that you normally use of the fact that you have a bitch whelping and it is often polite to inform the vet on duty when she goes into labour. He or she may then give you their advice on what best to do if you should become concerned. Sometimes veterinary practices might ask you to let the surgery know if ever an inter-birth interval exceeds a specified length of time, just so they are forewarned that you might be seeking further help and can prepare accordingly. Under such circumstances always make sure you let the surgery know if the bitch resumes whelping naturally.

THE THIRD STAGE OF WHELPING

The final stage of whelping is usually almost a continuation of the second stage and comprises the expulsion of the placenta (the 'afterbirth') once the puppy has been delivered. Placentas are not always expelled with each puppy. Sometimes they are retained and expelled later. Bitches will tend to eat the placentas as a natural behaviour and they can be so enthusiastic that they consume the placenta directly it passes through the vulva.

Try to keep a count of the placentas so you can be reassured that all have been passed and none retained after the bitch has finished whelping. However, placental retention is not necessarily a problem since, unless there is infection, any that remain will simply be resorbed within the uterus over time and cause no further problem.

Some people like to collect up these afterbirths rather than allow the bitch to eat them. This can be understandable since the sight of the bitch consuming the afterbirths can seem repulsive to some people and on occasion they cause the bitch to subsequently pass copious dark fluid faeces at a time when her house-training may lapse. However, this is a perfectly natural process and there is reason to believe that it can be beneficial

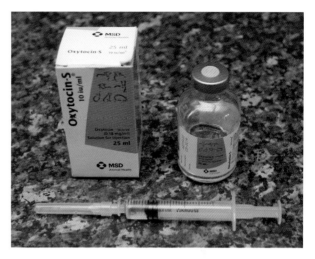

Oxytocin is normally given by deep intramuscular injection. It stimulates uterine contractions and can be used to assist whelping. Oxytocin injected once a bitch has finished whelping will help the uterus contract down, expel any retained afterbirths and stimulate milk let-down for the puppies.

to leave the bitch to consume at least some of her placentas because the afterbirth may contain substances that assist the uterus to close down.

Once your bitch appears to have finished whelping, settled down and started nursing her litter, leave her quietly for twenty-four hours and then have your vet check her over. This provides the vet an opportunity to ensure the uterus is empty and, if appropriate, give the bitch an injection of oxytocin. Oxytocin can be helpful at this point in time insofar as it will help expel anything left in the uterus, such as a retained placenta, and will stimulate the uterus to contract down completely.

NEO-NATAL CARE

Newborn puppies are relatively immature. The eyes and ears, for instance, are tightly closed at birth and only start to open at around ten to fourteen days of age. Puppies cannot maintain their body heat and are highly susceptible to cooling during the first few days of life. To maintain their body temperature, neo-natal puppies rely on lying on or near something warm, either their mother or the warmth you provide in the whelping box. This is why it is so important to site the whelping box somewhere warm where there are no draughts.

Many breeders suspend an infrared heat lamp above the whelping box and these can either be purchased from agricultural suppliers or are available from online retailers. Suspend the lamp on a chain and attach this to a hook above the box; the height of the lamp can then be adjusted simply by attaching a suitable link in the chain. It is much more important, however, to ensure that the puppies are nestling together in a nice warm box, and that you aren't just providing heat from above whilst they might be lying on a chilled surface; if necessary, electric heater pads are available that you can put under the bedding in one corner of the box.

Fleecy bedding material such as Vetbed or the equivalent is popular and suitable for the bitch and litter to lie on. This material has the advantage of allowing urine and other fluids to pass through whilst the surface remains dry, so put something absorbent underneath such as newspaper. Vetbed can be washed in a washing machine and is quick to dry. You will need to change the bedding regularly so by purchasing three suitably sized pieces of bedding you should always have at least one clean and available to use at any time.

Factors that are important in helping to ensure that newborn puppies survive will include:

- Ensuring you understand when the bitch is likely to whelp. The time of parturition should be estimated (blood sampling of progesterone levels prior to mating is especially helpful in this respect) so you are best able to monitor the bitch during the peri-natal period and the onset of parturition predicted by monitoring rectal temperature.
- Making sure there is someone on hand who is aware of the normal whelping process and will be able to recognize the various stages and any signs that the bitch may be having problems.
- The standard of hygiene in the whelping area. Thoroughly clean and disinfect the whelping box prior to occupancy and then wipe it over regularly and clean it as necessary to ensure that any surface the puppies come in contact with remains uncontaminated, fresh and dry.

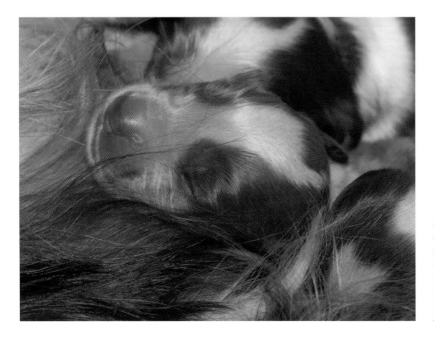

Neo-natal puppies are blind, deaf and unable to control their body temperature. They can, however, naturally seek out and find a nipple to feed from and thereafter snuggle up closely to the bitch and their littermates to sleep.

- Deciding on how closely to manage the whelping process and how much assistance to provide the bitch. If she has had a previous litter, experience may indicate whether she is able to whelp with little or no assistance, or whether some intervention may be appropriate. It is usually appropriate to 'whelp' the bitch, delivering and reviving each puppy by removing the placental attachments and foetal membranes, vigorously drying the pup to initiate respiration, and ensuring that each puppy suckles and receives adequate colostrum.

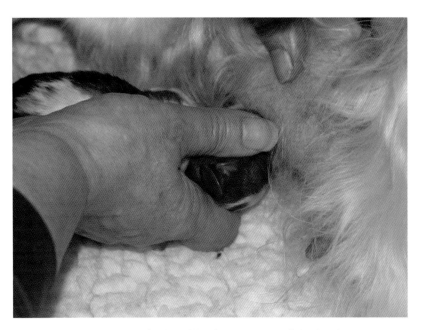

Assisting a newborn to find and latch on to one of the bitch's teats to ensure it suckles and consequently gets colostrum, the 'first milk', containing vital constituents like antibodies.

It is important for puppies to receive adequate colostrum (the first milk) from their mother during the first twelve to twenty-four hours of life. Colostrum contains antibodies to all the diseases that their mother has been exposed to or been vaccinated against, and it is important for them to have this temporary 'passive' immunity until they are old enough to be vaccinated.

It is helpful to weigh puppies at birth and check their weight regularly for the first week or so. Handling puppies like this is important for their future socialization, as is their exposure to mild aversive stimuli such as brief contact with a cool surface or a damp towel.

Healthy puppies are quiet, sleepy, warm to the touch, plump, round and firm. Occasionally they should make a

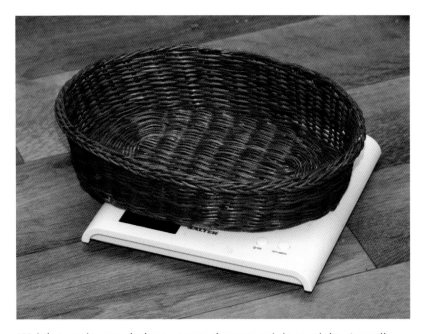

Weigh puppies regularly to ensure they are gaining weight. A small basket can be used to hold the puppy whilst you record the weight. Remember to weigh the basket first and then subtract that weight from the weight indicated by the scales in order to ascertain the weight of the puppy.

contented murmuring noise, and a sharp yelp if squashed or pushed off a teat.

The rectal temperature of a puppy at birth is normally 35.6–36.1°C, increasing gradually to 37.8°C by one week of age. During the first day of a puppy's life, the respiratory rate can range from eight to eighteen breaths per minute, depending on the size of the breed. Smaller breeds have a faster metabolic rate and so have correspondingly faster respiratory and heart rates. At two days of age, the respiratory rate increases to fifteen to thirty-five breaths per minute and by two weeks of age, twelve to thirty-five breaths per minute is the normal range. The heart rate of a newborn puppy can range from 120 to more than 180 beats per minute.

An unhealthy puppy will tend to isolate itself from its littermates and although it might nuzzle the bitch's teat, will not necessarily latch on and suckle properly. It will be limp when picked up, and will tend to have a wrinkled skin that is cold and clammy to the touch. The belly and feet are often bluish-purple in colour, the pup is likely to be lethargic and may utter a pathetic, plaintive cry or simply remain silent.

Any smaller puppies will benefit if you keep putting them on to a bitch's teat periodically through the first few days. Ensuring they get sufficient milk in this way, they should soon catch up, gain weight and soon look more like their larger littermates.

If a bitch continually rejects a puppy knowing instinctively that something is fundamentally wrong, and that her pup is unlikely to survive, you may be advised to have the pup humanely put to sleep at this early stage.

Puppies that are thriving well should gain weight steadily although the loss of an odd ounce or two one day is nothing to worry about, and they should double their birth weight in about seven days. Any that are small at birth should catch up rapidly once they are weaned.

Peri-natal and especially neo-natal losses are not necessarily unusual. Although precise figures are unobtainable, relatively conservative estimates rate losses as high as 15–30 per cent. These figures, taken in association with the fact that a proportion of embryos will not survive pregnancy, indicate the importance that should be placed on monitoring puppies through the first few hours and days of life in order to keep such losses to the absolute minimum. Veterinary opinion should always be sought for any unexplained deaths beyond the first seven-day period.

CONGENITAL AND DEVELOPMENTAL ABNORMALITIES

There are a variety of relatively common abnormalities that may either be apparent at birth, when they are known as 'congenital' abnormalities, or become apparent as the puppy grows and starts its early development, during the neonatal period. Many are simply points to be aware of, a few can be more serious, and most can be corrected if necessary as the dog matures.

So once the litter is established, the bitch has settled down and the puppies appear to be suckling vigorously, examine each puppy carefully for obvious signs of any congenital defects. It is good practice to have your vet check the litter, certainly if any are to be docked, and arrangements can normally be made either for a visit or for an appointment at the surgery in a manner that will minimize the risk of your young puppies being exposed to infection.

Cleft palate

This is seen as an abnormal mid-line opening in the roof of the mouth (the palate) and as a consequence there is an abnormal opening between the mouth and the nasal passage. In puppies it results from failure of the two sides of the palate to fuse together during embryonic development. In older dogs, accidental trauma to the roof of the mouth can also cause a cleft palate.

Unless obvious at birth, and it's always a good idea to check each pup as it's born for developmental abnormalities such as these, the first signs that a puppy may have a cleft palate will include:

- Difficulty sucking and nursing
- Breathing difficulties due to milk and food passing up into the nasal passage and entering the lungs

- Runny nose
- Coughing.

Puppies often develop an aspiration pneumonia resulting from milk and food particles entering the lungs and setting up infection. Later this will lead on to:

- Lack of appetite
- Slow growth
- Weight loss.

Cleft palate is most often a congenital disorder and is likely to be inherited because there are some breed predilections. Among the gundogs, Cocker Spaniels and Labrador Retrievers seem more affected although otherwise it is mainly seen in brachycephalic (short-nosed) breeds.

Cleft palate can also result from exposing pregnant bitches to various chemicals. Feeding excessively high levels of either vitamins A or B12 to pregnant bitches has been known to cause cleft palate in their puppies (never over-supplement pregnant bitches; good-quality rations contain all essential nutrients). There is also a risk from giving drugs like griseofulvin and corticosteroids to bitches during early pregnancy.

Puppies with cleft palate require intensive nursing. They will certainly need hand- if not tube-feeding and appropriate periodic antimicrobial drug therapy to treat any secondary aspiration pneumonia. Surgical closure of the opening is effective when carried out at six to eight weeks of age, before the general health of the puppy starts to become compromised, but only if the defect is small. More severe defects may need grafts or prosthetic implants for repair and often require multiple surgeries. Obviously there are ethical questions that need to be addressed in such cases and many would argue that such puppies are better to be humanely euthanized.

Umbilical hernia

An umbilical hernia is a condition in which abdominal contents protrude through the abdominal wall at the area of the umbilicus (the belly button). Umbilical hernias are most commonly a congenital malformation, so will be obvious at or

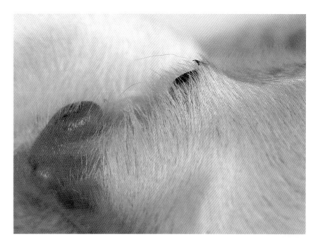

An umbilical hernia in a three-day-old puppy is seen as a swelling in the area where the umbilical cord was attached. In this case the hernia could be reduced and the abdominal contents, typically a small amount of fat, easily pushed back through the abdominal wall.

soon after birth. The umbilical opening contains blood vessels that pass through from the mother to the foetus as the umbilical cord. This opening then closes at birth in the normal dog and a hernia only results if the opening fails to close.

The hernia appears as a soft abdominal mass at the area of the umbilical ring and can usually be diagnosed by finding the swelling caused by the hernia on physical examination. Generally the contents of the hernia sack can be displaced back into the abdomen.

Depending on the size of the opening, abdominal structures (most commonly fat) can float into it. Generally this is of little significance and small hernias are generally not a problem. However, if the opening is large enough, a loop of intestines can descend through it, become strangulated and if left untreated, this can then become a life-threatening problem. It is recommended that you have your vet check any umbilical hernia to determine the size of the opening.

If a puppy has a small umbilical hernia, get into the habit of regularly pushing the contents back into the abdomen; your vet can show you how to do this if you are uncertain. The opening

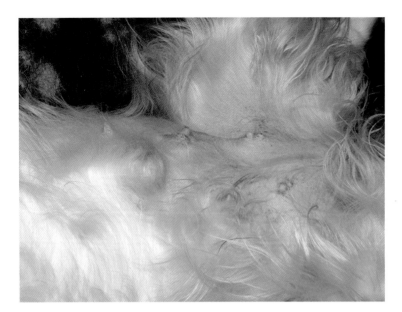

An umbilical hernia in an older bitch.

in the abdomen is essentially defective 'gristle' and will generally remain the same size as the dog grows progressively bigger to the point that, once mature, the opening is so relatively small as to allow little or nothing to pass through.

The exact cause of umbilical hernias is unknown although most are thought to be inherited, and for this reason it is generally recommended that dogs with umbilical hernias are not used for breeding. Interestingly some male dogs with umbilical herniation may also have a retained abdominal testicle.

Inguinal hernia

An inguinal hernia is a condition in which the abdominal contents protrude through the inguinal canal or inguinal ring, an opening that occurs in the muscle wall in the groin area. This is the canal through which the testes must descend in male puppies. Inguinal hernias occur more commonly in bitches. They may be classified as complicated or uncomplicated. A complicated hernia is one in which contents of the abdominal cavity have passed through the opening and become entrapped.

Most inguinal hernias are uncomplicated and cause no symptoms other than a swelling in the groin area. However, if contents from the abdom-inal cavity (such as the bladder or a loop of intestines) pass through the opening and become trapped, the situation can become more serious and potentially life threatening. Sometimes one or both horns of the uterus can pass through into the hernia and this would cause problems if the bitch became pregnant; certainly a bitch with an inguinal hernia should not be bred.

Cleft lip

Also referred to as 'hare lip' and more correctly as palatoschisis or congenital oronasal fistula, cleft lip is a defect that occurs when a puppy's lip or mouth does not form properly during early pregnancy. Cleft lip occurs if the tissue that makes up the lip does not join completely before birth. This results in an opening in the upper lip, which can be a very small slit or may be a large opening that extends into the nose. A puppy may be born with a cleft lip, a cleft palate, or with both a cleft lip and a cleft palate; these defects are called 'oro-facial clefts'.

Dentition

There are a variety of anomalies that can affect the teeth and jaws of dogs. Breeders will place a lot of emphasis on the mouth (the 'bite' as it is called) and show judges in particular will

The 'scissor' bite, shown in this dog skull, is the normal arrangement where the incisor teeth in the top and bottom jaw meet and are in contact to overlap those in the bottom jaw.

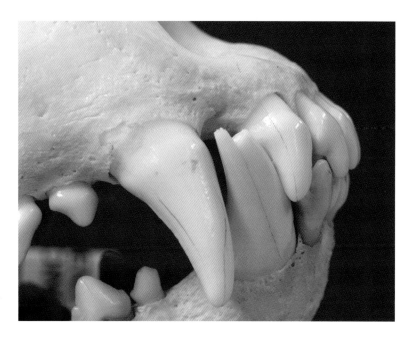

examine the front teeth to check for a correctly aligned bite. Fed an appropriate diet, domestic dogs will survive and thrive despite anomalously formed mouths, 'shovelling' food into their mouth and swallowing it direct rather than performing all the functions required of the various teeth in a wild canine. It is advisable, however, to be aware of what's normal and the terminology used to describe a number of the more common variations.

An adult dog should have forty-two teeth in total. Puppies are born with slightly fewer teeth, which they lose at around four to six months of age as their adult teeth erupt.

A 'scissor' bite is the normal arrangement where the incisor teeth in the top and bottom jaw meet and are in contact to overlap those in the bottom jaw. The result is a perfectly correct scissor arrangement that would enable the dog to grasp and tear flesh off a carcass.

A 'level' jaw is where the upper and lower incisors meet precisely and do not overlap. This is a minor point that appears to have little significance, however there is a possibility that as the dog ages and the teeth wear, the crown of the incisors will be subject to excess wear and subsequently expose the pulp cavity inside the tooth as the overlying enamel wears away.

A 'wry' mouth is a definite abnormality that can cause the dog potential discomfort and difficulty in eating. Here one mandible (lower jaw bone) is longer than the other causing gross misalignment of not only the teeth but also the jaws. The lower jaw will deviate to one side of

the mouth depending on which side the mandible is affected. If there is gross misalignment the defect may require surgical correction to provide the dog with at least some degree of normal function.

An 'overshot' jaw is one in which the length of the upper and lower jaws differ; the upper being longer than the lower.

An 'undershot' jaw is the opposite of an overshot jaw. Here the lower jaw is longer, sometimes such that the lower incisors protrude, giving the dog a 'bulldog face' appearance.

Obviously some breeds inherently have a tendency towards one or other of these anomalies in order to create the characteristic appearance of their head. Gundogs, however, should ideally have good mouths with a perfect scissor bite and be free of any of these defects.

Hydrocephalus

This is a condition in which excessive fluid is found within and around the brain. Hydrocephalus can occur as a result of trauma or a brain tumour, but here we are concerned only with the congenital condition that usually becomes apparent in young puppies of a few weeks of age and in older dogs up to a year of age.

Within the brain are fluid-filled spaces called ventricles. In a hydrocephalic dog, the ventricles fill with too much fluid. Congenital hydrocephalus arises when either the body produces too much cerebrospinal fluid or, as in most cases, the fluid that is produced cannot drain as it normally does from the central nervous system. The ventricles then become swollen, and the increased pressure damages and/or prevents development of the surrounding brain tissue. Toy breeds such as Maltese, Yorkshire Terriers, Pomeranians and Chihuahuas are most commonly affected although hydrocephalus can occur in other breeds as well.

Congenital hydrocephalus is usually diagnosed when the dog is young, usually less than four months of age, when the head takes on a dome-shaped appearance and the skull bones at the top of the head fail to close. A soft spot may be noticed on the top of the cranium (head) that is known as an 'open fontanel'. Affected puppies may be blind, have seizures or walk with an altered gait. Hydrocephalic dogs are often mentally dull and have a limited ability to learn. Different levels of severity exist but typically affected dogs have a very limited life span; few dogs with this condition live to be over two years of age.

Most cases go untreated because treatment is expensive and usually unsuccessful. Even with surgery and/or long-term medical treatment, the dog will rarely live a normal life.

Swimmer puppy syndrome

This is a term used to describe a puppy that is unable to stand, has a flattened chest and paddles his legs rather like a turtle. The condition is normally apparent in the first two weeks of life. Whereas normal puppies will be standing and walking by three weeks, swimmers are generally unable to stand at that age. Swimmer puppies occur more commonly in the dwarf (chondrodystrophic) breeds.

Unless some form of corrective therapy is instigated, due to their abnormally flattened chests swimmers tend to have poor circulation and suffer respiratory difficulties. Affected puppies can have difficulty swallowing and retaining food in their stomachs. They tend to be difficult and slow to wean (assuming they are able to survive to that stage) and are certainly unlikely to survive to the age of eight weeks.

Treatment typically comprises taping the legs in the correct position. If this is done early enough, as soon as the condition is recognized and diagnosed, you should see almost immediate progress. Swimming sessions, three times daily, will also help by building muscle. Submerge the puppy up to its chin in water where its survival instinct will induce it to kick its legs and exercise its muscles.

Since there may be a hereditary component to this condition, dogs that were swimmers as puppies should not be bred.

OTHER DEVELOPMENTAL ABNORMALITIES

Unless gross, any other developmental abnormalities will only become apparent as the puppy matures during the later pre-wean period. These include such abnormalities as a kinked tail, or screw-tail; the former will not usually cause any problems but will render the puppy unsuitable for showing. Screw-tail (unless it occurs in a breed such as the Bulldog where it is normal to have such a tail) is often more significant because it can indicate external evidence of spinal deformity.

Think carefully about how you are going to deal with any such issues and take the advice of your vet concerning the immediate situation and any likely long-term effects so that you can decide on an appropriate course of action that will be in the best interests of the puppy. Whilst undershot puppies will be perfectly suitable as pets, you might decide, for instance, that it might be more humane to allow the vet to euthanize a puppy with hydrocephalus.

BREATHING PROBLEMS

Breathing problems in puppies are quite common and occur for a variety of reasons. They are not always serious, but they do need to be identified. Always keep a close eye on a puppy that is exhibiting any sign of difficulty breathing and seek veterinary opinion if it persists.

There are different types of breathing problems; each is unique to the puppy and its environment and some are hereditary. These problems generally cause the puppy to have laboured breathing. It may snore continuously whilst asleep, or pant in a way that does not correspond with its level of activity. Obviously those seen in short-nosed brachycephalic breeds are due entirely to the anatomy of the dog; these puppies will generally have more laboured breathing after exercise, which should subside within thirty minutes. Other conditions may be more serious and need immediate treatment.

A dog that suffers from breathing problems for more than twenty-four hours, despite behaving normally otherwise, should be seen by a veterinarian. If the puppy seems to be in pain or is non-responsive, it should be taken to a vet immediately. While some breathing problems will resolve on their own, more serious ones may need to be treated with antibiotics or require surgery. If in any doubt, it's better to seek professional advice and if your vet can find no obvious cause then it is likely that the problem will resolve in time; often as the puppy gets older, as the shape of the head alters and the nose gets longer.

NOTES ON BOTTLE-FEEDING PUPPIES

It is relatively unusual for a bitch to be unable to rear her puppies. If a particular puppy is being rejected by the bitch there is a very good chance that it is unhealthy, that she is aware of this, and that this is the reason she is rejecting it. Even though you may find nothing wrong there is a good chance that you will not succeed in hand-rearing the puppy.

Much of the advice given here also applies to supplemental feeding that may be required if the bitch does not have sufficient milk for a large litter, or if a smaller puppy requires a little extra, or if one or two puppies are being pushed aside by their more robust littermates. This is a little easier than hand-rearing an entire litter with no assistance from the bitch.

Hand-rearing a litter of puppies is labour intensive and can be a daunting task. It requires considerable time and dedication. If you are placed in the situation of having to rear puppies by hand you should contact your veterinary practice for advice and try to make sure you have people who are willing to help and support you. The intensive feeding schedule is tiring and cleaning up and monitoring the litter is time-consuming. Helpers can make a big difference.

The following equipment is recommended:

- Syringes – 2ml for puppies
- Rearing bottle(s) available from your vet, online or your local pet shop
- Teats – assorted sizes are available depending on the size of the puppy
- Cotton wool
- A room thermometer
- Another thermometer to measure the temperature of the milk prior to feeding
- Weighing scales – to weigh the puppies each day. The scales will need to weigh accurately to the nearest 1–5g
- Milton Sterilising Fluid – equipment should be sterilized and stored without rinsing, then rinsed thoroughly just prior to use.

Equipment should be kept very clean, and milk should be made up daily and kept in the fridge (ready to warm up for each feed).

As hand-rearing is very demanding, and bitches generally rear litters of puppies better than any person, consider the possibility of finding a foster mother. This is not always easy and your enquiries may not be successful. Ask your veterinary practice in the first instance, as they may know of a bitch with puppies of similar age or one that is heavily in milk from having concurrent pseudopregnancy. Pet forums on social media and breed clubs are other areas of enquiry. One big advantage of a foster mother is that the bitch can teach the puppies things that humans cannot, like learning bite inhibition.

Puppies require colostrum, a highly concentrated mixture of antibodies and other nutrients, present in bitch's milk produced during the first twenty-four hours after whelping. Most litters are hand-reared after this time so will have received colostrum, but if the puppies have been deprived of it your vet may be able to administer oral or injectable doses of blood serum or plasma from a healthy dog to compensate. Puppies that have not received colostrum are more vulnerable to infection and illness.

The bitch stimulates her puppies to urinate and defecate, so in her absence this becomes your job. You'll need a supply of cotton wool pads and some luke-warm water to gently massage the area around the anus and urinary orifice after every feed. Don't be concerned if urination or defecation doesn't happen every time. Monitor the colour and consistency of the puppies' stools; their faeces are normally a little sticky, but if they become loose, seek veterinary advice promptly because young puppies can soon become dehydrated and lose electrolytes if they develop diarrhoea. Once the litter is about three weeks old, the pups should be urinating and defecating by themselves; they will just require a little help cleaning themselves up afterwards.

Recommended milk substitutes:

- Welpi – which is especially formulated for puppies
- Pedigree Instant Milk Substitute – again, a special puppy formula
- Lactol – a milk substitute but not species specific
- Lamblac – a ewes' milk substitute, only suitable for supplementary feeding puppies.

It is essential to make up and use milk substitutes in accordance with the manufacturers' instructions. Milk substitute should be made up fresh for each feed and warmed to 38°C (body temperature) before feeding. Formula milk especially for puppies is the best option, and it makes life much easier as you simply add water.

Puppies should increase their bodyweight by 5–10 per cent per day for the first two weeks of life (although it is normal for them to lose weight in the first day of life and, again, after the removal of dewclaws or following tail docking). Failure to grow at this rate may indicate underfeeding or ill health. It is helpful to weigh each puppy every day and to keep a record so you can check to make sure that all the puppies are growing well. Weigh your puppies at the same time each day, for example after a particular feed, and note whether or not they have urinated and/or defecated beforehand.

The milk should be warmed to body temperature and fed using a special feeding bottle with a teat from which the puppy can suckle. However, you may find it easier to use a syringe with a teat attached for the first week of life unless the puppies have a good, vigorous suckling reflex. Nursing bottles are not recommended until the puppy has a strong, well-developed suckling reflex. Take care syringe feeding because aspiration pneumonia (where milk is inhaled into the lungs rather than going down into the stomach) is more of a risk when using this method.

Puppies should be fed on their stomachs, not upright or upside-down, and the head must not be over-extended. It is very important that you feed puppies very slowly, keeping their heads up to allow them to swallow. If you give milk too fast it might go down the wrong way (into the airways), which could lead to pneumonia.

If you are attempting to save a weak puppy it is best to feed it with a stomach tube rather than giving milk substitute by mouth. This should be carried out by someone who is competent and suitably trained as it involves passing a tube through the mouth, down the throat and into the stomach. Milk is then placed into a syringe and injected down the tube. A veterinary nurse will often be pleased to demonstrate how to stomach-feed the puppies initially.

Make sure you are feeding suitable volumes according to the instructions for the puppies' age and weight, and don't be tempted to over-feed them, as again this can result in aspiration pneumonia or cause diarrhoea.

Feed every two hours until the pups are a week old (although you can sometimes leave them from 12pm until 4am if the pups are not underweight). Feeds can be reduced to four-hourly for the second week. From three weeks of age, six-hourly feeds are generally suitable. Much will depend on the individual litter, and some pups may need more frequent feeding. At four weeks of age, the normal four feeds per day are usually acceptable. Puppies can be weaned at three to four weeks of age when liquidized solid food can start to be gradually introduced.

Puppies are unable to properly regulate their body temperature until they are two weeks of age and prior to this they cannot generate enough heat to keep themselves warm. Conse-quently they should be kept warm but not too hot. The ambient temperature of their accommodation should be in the region of 29–30°C. If your puppies get too cold, warm them up slowly. The ambient temperature can then gradually be reduced, so by the time they are four weeks of age, they can be kept at normal room temperature. Ideally the humidity level should be at about 55–65 per cent; if the atmosphere is too dry it can contribute to the puppies becoming dehydrated.

5 RAISING THE LITTER

In this chapter we will be focussing on the litter, following the puppies from early neo-natal life through periods when they begin to develop their independence and individual personalities to the point where they are prepared to leave for their new homes.

THE NEO-NATAL PERIOD

Once the litter is whelped and established, all the puppies should be suckling well and be taking in their colostrum. It is important that puppies receive adequate colostrum from their mother during the first twelve to twenty-four hours of life. Colostrum contains antibodies to all the diseases that their mother has been exposed to or been vaccinated against and it is important for them to be protected by this temporary passive immunity until they are old enough to be vaccinated.

Puppies are born blind and deaf but have their senses of touch, taste and smell, most of which will be directed towards finding the milk bar and suckling. The puppies will normally settle into a routine of feeding, being cleaned up by the bitch, and sleeping.

Newborn puppies are relatively immature, cannot maintain their body heat and rely on lying on

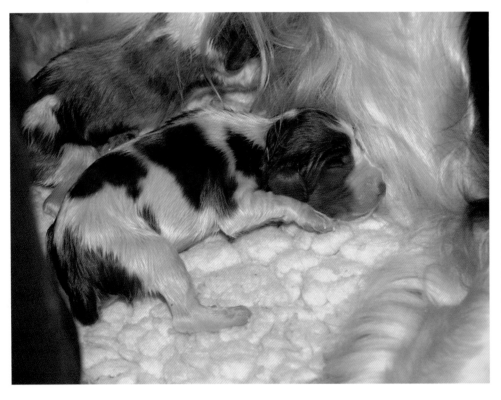

A newborn puppy that has been revived, encouraged to suckle, taken its first milk feed and settled down to sleep whilst the bitch prepares to give birth to another puppy. Born blind and deaf, the eyes and the entrances to the ear canals will not normally open until they are ten to fourteen days of age.

or near something warm, either their mother or the warmth you provide in the whelping box. The eyes and ears are tightly closed and only begin to open around ten to fourteen days of age.

It is helpful to weigh puppies at birth and then check their weight regularly for the first week or so. Handling puppies is important for their future socialization, as is their exposure to mild aversive stimuli such as brief contact with a cool surface or a damp towel.

Healthy puppies are quiet, sleepy, warm to the touch, plump, round and firm. Occasionally they will twitch and should make contented murmuring noises, and a sharp yelp if squashed or pushed off a teat.

The behaviour of the bitch towards her pups should be observed; first-time whelpings and nervous or insecure bitches may require least disturbance to allow them to settle down and calm their litter. Some inexperienced bitches may require assistance to clean their pups and, by licking them, stimulate the puppies to pass urine and faeces.

Puppies instinctively move towards the teat and will latch on to suckle; know the signs that indicate that the bitch's milk is flowing and that every puppy in the litter is suckling successfully. Puppies that are suckling well make paddling movements and will often raise their tail, as a characteristic reflex, when first expressing and ingesting milk from the teat.

The whelping box should be wiped over regularly and cleaned as necessary to ensure that any surface the puppies come in contact with remains uncontaminated, fresh and dry.

In my experience, with appropriate management, the overall level of neo-natal losses with-

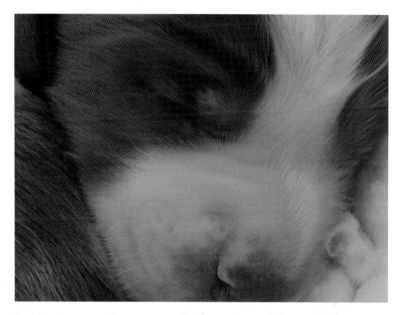

By the time puppies are a week of age they will have developed obvious eyelids in preparation for their eyes to open.

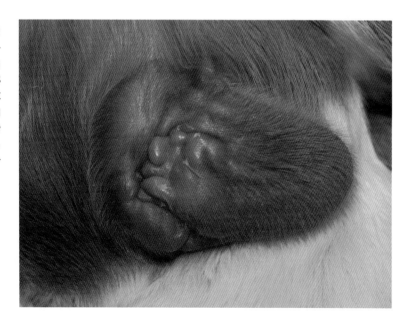

The opening to the external ear canal is closed in neo-natal puppies.

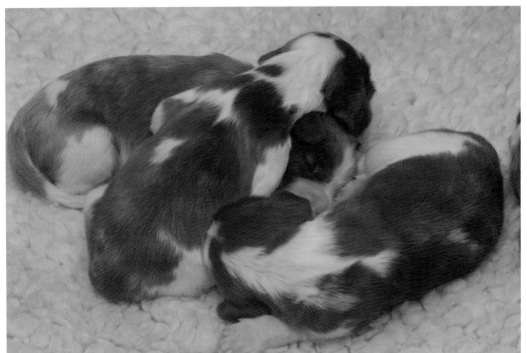

In the absence of the bitch, neo-natal puppies will customarily huddle up together and go to sleep.

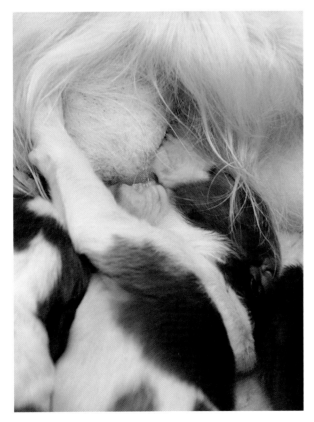

When latched on to a teat, the puppy should have a strong suckling reflex and it should take some effort to overcome the suction of suckling and remove a puppy from its teat. The pups will paw each side of the teat to stimulate milk let-down and push themselves up and on to the teat with their hind feet.

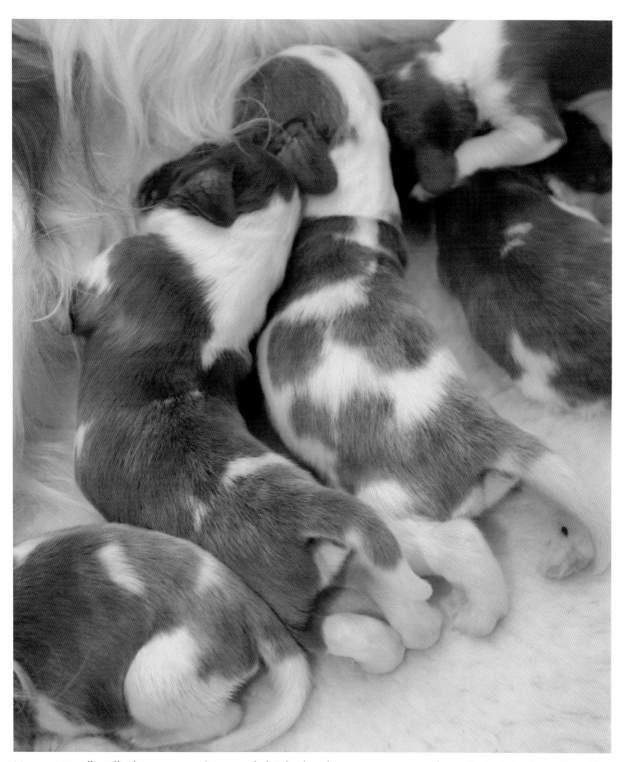

You can usually tell when a puppy is properly latched on because as soon as the milk starts to flow, the tail will stiffen and rise.

in a breeding kennel (the proportion of pups born alive that do not survive the first three days of life) can be reduced to as little as 5–7 per cent.

During the immediate three-day post-whelp period the bitch will be reluctant to leave her puppies, but thereafter may choose to leave the litter for progressively longer periods. Give your bitch short periods of gentle exercise at this time.

Dewclaws

These can be removed at three to four days of age. The dewclaw is the equivalent of the puppy's thumb; a fifth digit, generally regarded as serving little purpose albeit in some particular breeds it is customary to retain the dewclaws. Increasingly I find people are inclined to leave dewclaws on the front feet and remove any that are loosely attached on the hind legs. This is probably to be recommended. If you examine footprints left in soft ground from a dog turning at any speed, you will often notice the imprint of the dewclaw so it certainly serves some purpose and might hardly be regarded as being redundant in (only) domestic canines. Do not be surprised if your puppies lose a little weight during the first twenty-four hours after having their dewclaws removed, but this should be no more than a few grams and should quickly be regained.

Docking of dog's tails

If the puppies are of a breed where it is customary to legally dock those used for work then this is best done once the litter is established at around three days of age, before the tail and any dewclaws that are to be removed become too substantial. The operation must be carried out by a veterinary surgeon, who should provide you a certificate accordingly. You can try to minimize any discomfort for the pups by applying a local anaesthetic such as Emla Cream, which is available from good chemists and can be bought without a prescription. Rub the cream well into the skin of the tail or dewclaws about twenty minutes prior to the operation. This won't make the procedure painless but is often sufficient to numb the skin whilst the incision is made.

ONE TO THREE WEEKS OF AGE

Neo-natal puppies are unable to support their weight and simply crawl around using paddling motions, mainly with their front legs. This limited movement, however, provides the exercise that develops muscle strength and limb coordination – very soon the puppies are crawling over and around each other and their mother.

Puppies that are thriving well should gain weight steadily although the loss of an odd

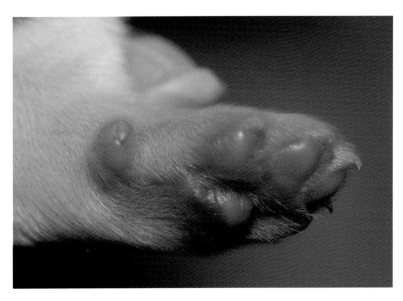

The dewclaw, on the left, on the hind foot of a three- to four-day-old puppy.

At seven days of age, puppies should be able to pull themselves up and move around on their forelegs. Some will even begin to get up on all four feet and take a few steps.

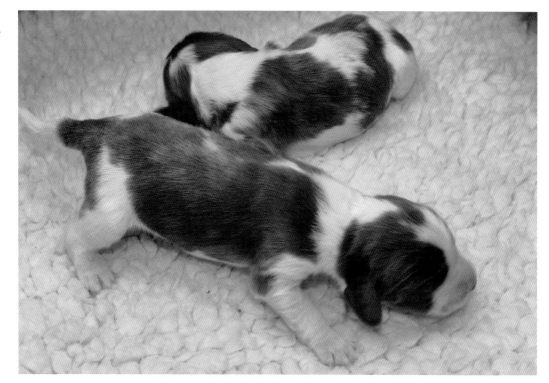

At seven to ten days of age, puppies will have developed very obvious eyelids and soon the eyes will just start to open.

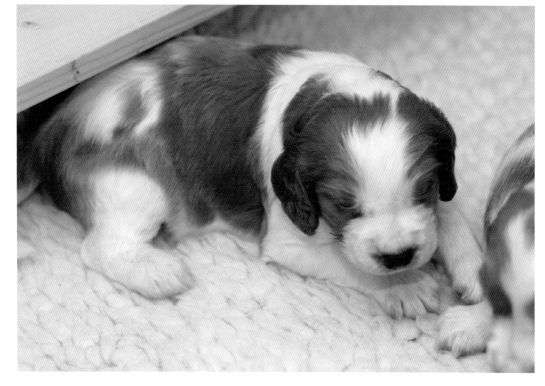

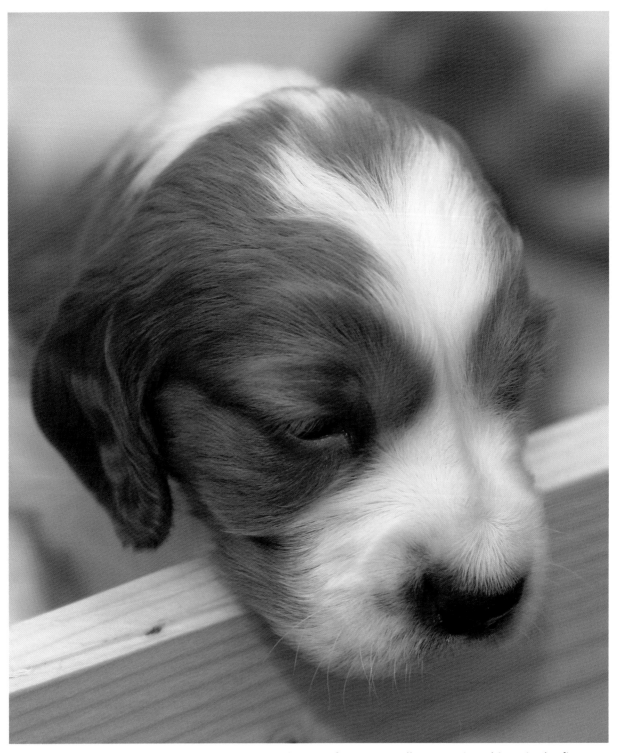

Once the eyes have opened the puppy will start to learn to focus, normally on moving objects in the first instance.

ounce or two one day is nothing to worry about, and they should double their birth weight in about seven days. Any that are small at birth should catch up rapidly once they are weaned. Losses beyond this first seven-day period should be low, < 5 per cent. Always seek your vet's opinion should any puppy die unexpectedly.

The second week brings great changes for the puppies. They will look plumper and stronger, and their faces will change so they look a little more dog-like.

Ears and eyes will start to open during this period. The ears should be open at about two weeks of age. Eyelids should start developing around seven to ten days of age and the eyes open by fourteen to sixteen days. This means they start to develop a sense of their world. They start to focus and learn what their mother and their littermates look and sound like. The puppies will begin to develop their own vocabulary and progress from mews to yelps, whines and even barking. Puppies can generally stand by two weeks of age and by three weeks will start to walk.

Once the pups are well established and more independent, normally at approximately ten to fourteen days of age, the bitch will frequently choose to leave her puppies, returning periodically to feed and care for them. From this point in time more extended periods of exercise can resume; just make sure she doesn't come in contact with any other dogs that are likely to represent an infection risk to your puppies, and don't take her to exercise in areas frequented by other dogs.

By three weeks of age, puppy development advances to a transitional period. This is a time of rapid physical and sensory development, during which the puppies go from total dependence on their mother to starting to become more independent. Puppy teeth begin to erupt. Puppies begin to play and otherwise interact with their littermates, to explore and learn about their environment and begin sampling food. At this stage the bitch will stop cleaning them up and the puppies should be able to intentionally defecate and void urine on their own. By this stage they should be able to see and hear quite well and you should see that

they recognize you when you approach their pen.

Continue to feed the bitch a high-quality diet in much the same way as through pregnancy (*see* Chapter 2). Producing sufficient milk to feed a large litter will take a lot out of a bitch and it is not uncommon for them to lose a little condition. As long as the bitch is feeding well and consuming an adequate diet, this should soon be regained once the litter is weaned, but whilst actively lactating do watch for signs of eclampsia (*see* below).

POST-PARTURIENT HEALTH CONCERNS FOR THE BITCH

Metritis

This is inflammation of the endometrium (the lining of the uterus/womb) due to bacterial infection, usually seen within a week of the bitch giving birth. It can be due to a number of potential causes such as a difficult birth or a prolonged delivery, or perhaps a large litter requiring obstetric manipulation. It also occurs in association with retained foetuses or placentas.

The bacteria that are most often responsible for metritis are those like Escherichia coli, which often spread into the bloodstream causing bacteraemia and toxaemia. Infection may lead on to sterility, and if untreated may prove to be fatal.

Metritis should be suspected if you see a green, foul-smelling discharge from the vulva, any purulent vaginal discharge, or a discharge of pus mixed with blood. The bitch is likely to be lethargic, off her food, producing less milk and generally showing signs of becoming a poor mother.

Always seek veterinary attention if you see any of these signs. Your veterinary surgeon may perform a number of tests to help determine whether the bacterial infection has spread to the bloodstream and collect a sample of the discharge for cytological (microscopic) examination. A culture of the discharge will help identify which bacteria are causing the infection and a sensitivity of the isolated bacteria may be used to determine the most appropriate antibiotic treatment.

The bitch may need to be hospitalized for more

intensive treatment, especially if she is septicae-mic. If the metritis is not too advanced, she will most likely respond to medical treatment. If no further breeding is planned, she may need to be spayed and certainly this will be appropriate if the metritis is secondary to retained foetuses or placentas, and when the uterus has ruptured, or is severely infected.

Eclampsia

Also referred to as either hypocalcaemia or puer-peral tetany, this is a life-threatening emergency medical condition associated with a precipitous drop in blood calcium that occurs in nursing bitches. Eclampsia is most commonly seen in bitches nursing puppies that are one to five weeks of age, a time when the bitch is having to produce most milk.

Eclampsia is not due to an overall lack of cal-cium and hence calcium supplementation for pregnant and nursing dogs is not recommend-ed. Providing excess calcium during pregnancy or lactation suppresses parathyroid hormone production and the net effect is an increased risk of eclampsia. The signs of eclampsia indicate that the nursing female simply cannot mobilize a sufficient amount of the calcium stored in her body quickly enough to meet the demands of her growing litter.

Bitches that develop eclampsia tend to be good mothers that are particularly attentive to their puppies. The signs include muscle tremors, weakness and a form of paralysis called puer-peral tetany. The latter is characterized by stiff limbs and an inability to stand or walk. The bitch may become very restless and/or start panting a lot, and you may notice that she is moving stiffly. Unless treated these signs can progress to mus-cle spasms affecting the whole body, which can quickly progress to convulsions.

Eclampsia is considered a medical emergency. If you suspect eclampsia is developing, prevent the pups from suckling and contact your veteri-nary surgeon immediately.

Treatment involves the intravenous administra-tion of calcium, which has to be given very care-fully and slowly. If the bitch is having seizures and tetany, the vet may also give anti-seizure drugs.

Once the condition is treated and the immediate signs are controlled the bitch will subsequently require oral calcium supplements and you will be recommended to wean the puppies as quickly as possible. A complete recovery from eclampsia is usually rapid if the condition is diagnosed soon enough.

Mastitis

An infection and inflammation of the mammary glands, mastitis is extremely painful for the bitch and may cause a variety of signs and symptoms. There are a number of possible causes although it is normally due to the bitch's teats becoming sore and cracking allowing bacteria, normally present on the skin, to enter the milk canal and multiply. Infection then spreads throughout the mammary tissue.

It is important to be aware of mastitis when a bitch is nursing a litter because as it can be painful, she can become irritable and refuse to allow the puppies to suckle. Consequently, the first sign of mastitis may be puppies unable to feed, when you may hear them constantly cry-ing and appearing lethargic. You will notice the mammary glands are hot, swollen, painful and hard to the touch. The bitch may also be off her food, depressed, disinterested in her puppies and have a foul-smelling discharge from her teats. In severe cases the mammary glands may absces-sate and rupture.

If you suspect mastitis seek the advice of your veterinary surgeon as soon as possible. This may require an out-of-hours call because any restric-tion in feeding the puppies can be potentially life threatening. Generally an experienced vet-erinary surgeon will be able to diagnose mastitis on physical examination.

Treatment depends upon the severity of the infection. In early cases a course of antibiotics may be sufficient; always complete the course of treatment even if it appears that the mastitis has cleared up. You may also be advised to apply warm compresses to the affected teats to relieve congestion and encourage the flow of milk. If the milk supply is compromised you may have to hand-feed the puppies until the mammary glands are free from infection.

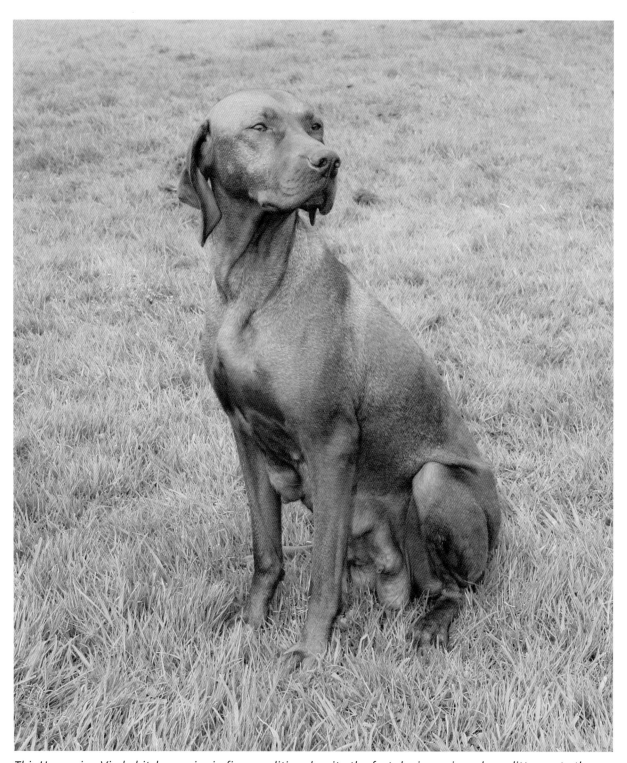

This Hungarian Vizsla bitch remains in fine condition despite the fact she is nursing a large litter; note the prominent mammary glands.

WEANING

Weaning is a term used to describe the process whereby there is a gradual reduction of a puppy's dependency on its mother's milk and care. It involves a progressive introduction to eating solid food and an associated and complementary withdrawal of the bitch so that her milk supply gradually dries up. In the wild, weaning begins naturally as soon as the puppies start to develop their teeth at three to four weeks of age. Natural weaning involves the female dog regurgitating her food and the puppies consuming this material. Many pet bitches will also regurgitate food for their puppies. This is a natural maternal function and nothing to necessarily be worried about. Many owners will tend to discourage it because it limits the amount of food available to the bitch and she will tend to lose more condition whilst nursing her litter as a consequence. Most puppies will be weaned and completely independent of their mother's milk by the age of six weeks or less. The overall intention is that they are fully weaned by the time they are ready to leave for their new homes, typically around eight weeks of age.

Weaning, when they start to consume solid food, can commence by offering some minced meat or puppy meal at around two to three weeks of age. Understand that puppies are able to take solid food before they are able to lap, albeit their consumption of solid feed can be somewhat messy at first but the bitch will usually clean them up.

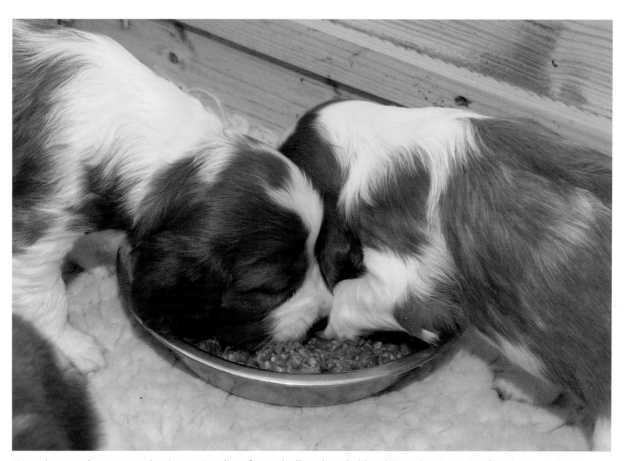

Weaning can be a messy business. Feeding from shallow bowls like this makes it easier for the puppies to access and ingest their food.

Once the puppies are eating solid food, start taking the bitch away periodically to encourage her milk to dry up and start giving them frequent small meals. Feed four meals daily, alternating a 'solid' meal of mince and puppy meal or a soaked complete feed, with 'milk' meals of milk, goat's milk, infant baby rice and so on. The bitch will now cease cleaning up her puppies, spend less and less time with them and eventually only want to visit them for relatively brief periods. Allow her to sleep in the same room as her puppies, but in a bed away from them that the litter cannot reach. Her milk should gradually dry up but if puppies continue to suckle this may make her sore and susceptible to mastitis, recognized as hard swellings within the mammary glands that are warm and painful to the touch. As the pups get older and larger they will make active attempts to leave the whelping box. Once they do, move them to a puppy pen or somewhere that you have set aside where the litter is safely enclosed with room to run around and grow on, separate from their mother and any other dogs you may have in the household. Provide them a variety of stimulating objects to play with, chew and tear up.

Ample space and these resources encourage the development of natural behaviours, including social behaviours such as play fighting. You now need to start socializing the puppies. Have them somewhere like the kitchen where they can become accustomed to the usual household smells, sounds and activities. Encourage visitors but not with other dogs. Try to make sure the pups are exposed to a variety of stimuli and experiences. Have people pick them up, cuddle and stroke them and as they get older try to ensure your puppies meet children and older people. Let the puppies out regularly, especially after meals, and this will encourage house-training, particularly if you make a point of praising the puppy as the deed is done.

BEHAVIOURAL DEVELOPMENT AND THE IMPORTANCE OF SOCIALIZATION

If puppies are not properly socialized they are likely to suffer a variety of behavioural disorders and develop into adult dogs that tend to be timid, intolerant and develop socially unacceptable patterns of behaviour. Behavioural disorders are not uncommon among the general dog population and constitute as much of a problem as many of the clinical diseases that vets have to treat. Poorly socialized dogs account for the vast majority of dogs that have to be destroyed at their owners' request because they cannot cope with their pet's behaviour.

Evidence from behavioural studies demonstrates that there is a 'window of opportunity', a prime socialization period, that starts at around three weeks of age and ends when the puppy reaches the age of sixteen weeks. During this period the puppy needs to be exposed to as wide a range of environmental stimuli as possible so that it will develop into a calm, well-socialized individual that is easy to train and able to cope with and tolerate a wide range of situations and circumstances.

As part of this early socialization, puppies should become accustomed to meeting strange people, other dogs and to loud, unexpected, noises. Socialization will also encourage them to start exploring confidently and ensuring that they do not become timid in strange surroundings.

Although puppies need to avoid being exposed to a variety of infectious diseases until they are fully vaccinated, there is no reason why during this period they cannot become accustomed to entering a vehicle so that later when they are old enough, their new owners can start taking them on short journeys. Bear in mind that in the country, where there are few strange dogs, other than avoiding places where there is likely to be vermin the risk of infection is far lower than, say, taking a new puppy to a communal urban park where other dogs are routinely exercised.

Encourage people to visit and meet your puppies but don't overwhelm them and don't allow people to bring their dogs with them. Try to make sure that the litter meets and interacts with children and older people and learns to behave accordingly. All such early experience is useful; remember that a dog's mental health is as important as its clinical health. It needs to be

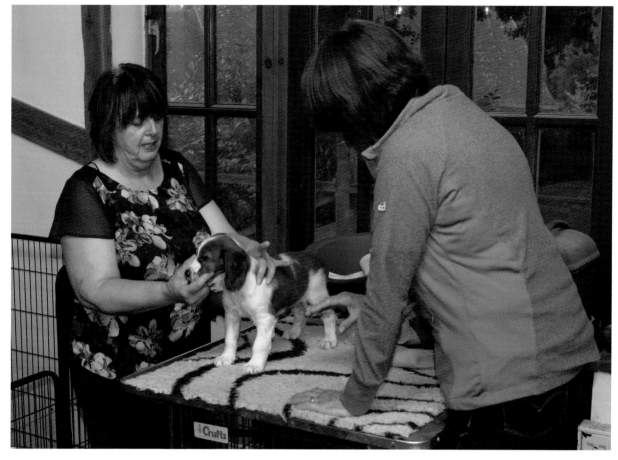

Having people, including friends and relations, visit to see your puppies is an excellent opportunity to help with socializing your litter. Puppies can be handled, restrained and examined in a controlled environment where you should ensure the puppy is as calm and relaxed as possible at all times.

fit in mind as well as fit and healthy in body, in other words fit to function as a pet or as a working dog, becoming socially acceptable, tolerant and obedient.

Commonly encountered problems in poorly socialized dogs include a fear of sudden loud noises, what's known as 'separation anxiety', where a dog cannot cope with being left on its own, difficulty entering and travelling in vehicles and timidity towards strangers, both human and canine. Getting a puppy accustomed to riding in a car is best done in stages. You can start at around six to eight weeks of age by first getting the puppies used to entering and sitting calmly in

a stationary car. Later start the engine and even, if all is well, move off.

Introduce your puppies to strange sights, sounds and smells and ensure they start to meet different types of people at the earliest opportunity. For instance, take advantage of occasions when potential new owners visit to see the litter as one obvious means by which your puppies can start to meet strangers. Ensure they are somewhere that they know to be safe when first meeting strangers. Make sure the puppies meet a cross-section of the population, not just close family members and friends of your age. They are likely to meet a wide range of people once they

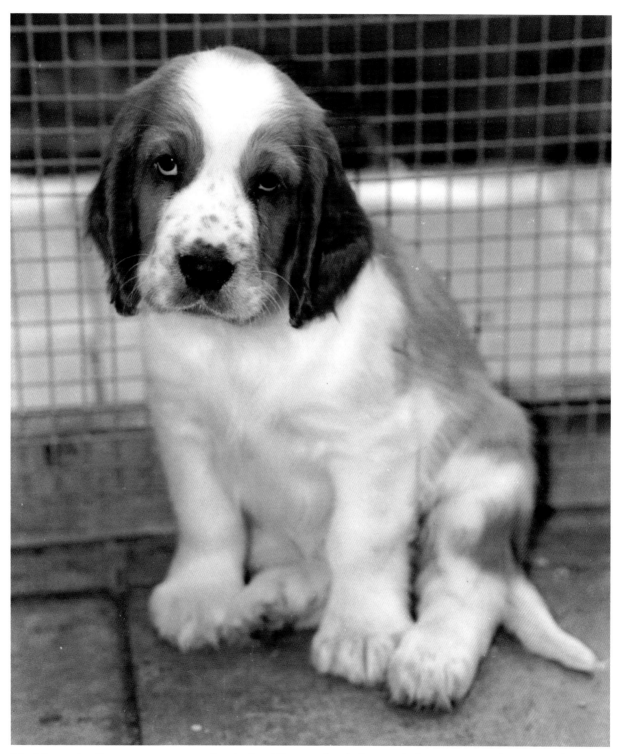

Most importantly, ensure your puppies start getting used to being on their own on occasions, away from their littermates.

are older so now is the time to start introducing your puppies to members of society in general. If you have the opportunity get them accustomed to meeting, for instance, people wearing bright clothing, young children, people wearing spectacles and sunglasses, people with beards and hats, and older people.

Whilst you may not be able to take your puppies out until fully vaccinated, don't shut the puppies away in a kennel or leave them alone in the puppy pen for longer than is necessary during the day. Try to provide an environment that best provides stimulatory opportunities. Many people tend to raise their litter in the kitchen because this is where there is most human activity as well as strange noises and vibrations from domestic appliances such as washing machines and vacuum cleaners. It is also one of the most practical places to bring up puppies, with floors that are easier to clean up after the odd 'accident' and tends to be the place where many people will feed their puppy and wash up food bowls afterwards. Banging pots and pans will help acclimatize the puppy to sudden unexpected noise and some owners deliberately use metal food bowls so that a puppy learns to associate noise with pleasant experiences.

It will be useful to let the puppies see you using long-handled implements such as mops, brooms and garden tools. Ensure they become used to seeing people using tools and other noisy appliances and that they don't become anxious, but are relaxed and not frightened or nervous in such situations.

Always greet your puppies when you return after leaving them on their own and when they are older, make a fuss of individual puppies in such a way that they start to learn a 'controlled greeting', meaning they don't become too excited when their owner(s) return. Again, when they are old enough, let the puppies out immediately to relieve themselves. This will assist with house-training and encourage your puppies to get into the habit of emptying their bladders on your return.

IMPORTANT: Always be very aware of the puppy and that he is having a good time. If he looks worried in any way, take it more slowly. Each puppy must be treated as an individual – and all this socialization and habituation has to be fun and rewarding for him.

If the puppy is very distressed when left, try using a DAP (dog appeasing pheromone) preparation available from your vet or online. DAP mimics the odour exuded by the dam and has a calming effect on puppies. It can also be used in other circumstances where you wish to avoid a puppy becoming too distressed, such as when first travelling in the car.

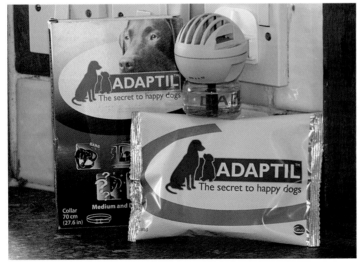

Dog appeasing pheromone (DAP) is available in a variety of forms suitable for use in various circumstances.

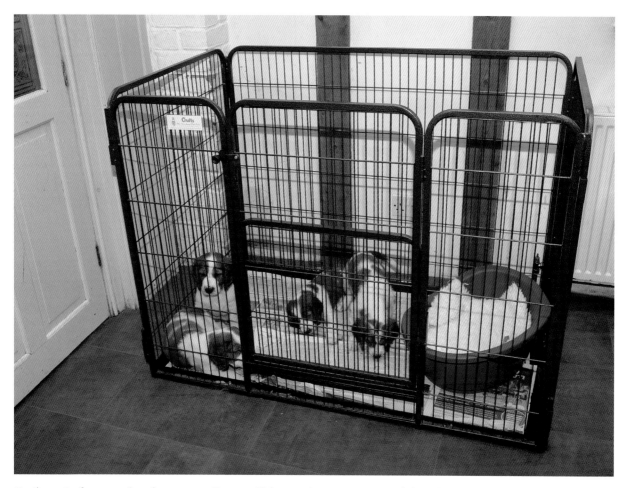

By three to four weeks of age most litters will be ready to move out of the whelping box and into a larger, more secure area where the puppies have more room to move around and start interacting with their littermates.

THREE TO FOUR WEEKS OF AGE

This is the point in time when, once the puppies are eating solid food and particularly after they have been wormed, the bitch will cease to clean up after them; this now becomes your job!

Given the opportunity most bitches will continue to regurgitate food for their puppies, which is not necessary once they start to consume some solid food and will simply deprive her of nutrients and tend to make her lose condition unnecessarily, so keep her away from the litter for about an hour after she has been fed.

This is a good time to move the litter out of the seclusion afforded by the whelping box and into a place where the puppies can start to see and explore a wider environment and where they can be better observed so you can monitor their subsequent development.

Within this new environment the litter should be provided with a separate place to sleep and a confluent exercise area in which they can defecate and urinate so as not to soil their bedding. Some people choose to provide a covered sleeping area – a large, stout cardboard box might suffice – which offers a suitable 'retreat' in which a puppy can lie quietly, away from its littermates, if it might prefer and/or choose to do so.

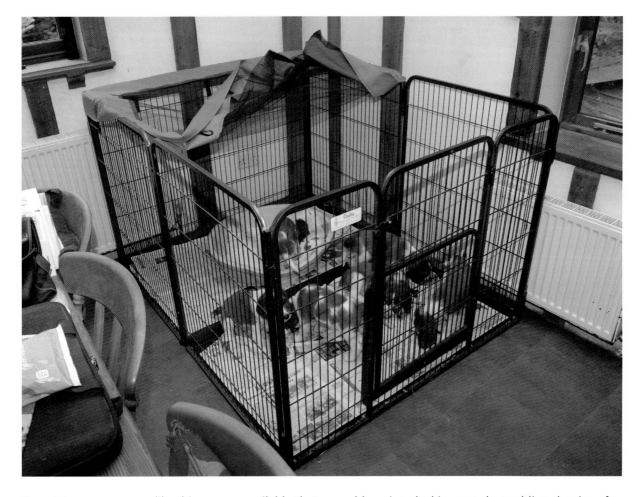

Proprietary puppy pens like this one are available that assemble as interlocking panels, enabling the size of the pen to be tailored to suitably accommodate various sizes of litters. The pen can also be enlarged as the puppies mature to provide additional space.

The puppy pen will typically comprise a secure enclosure where they won't accidentally injure themselves. In a domestic environment many people will opt to partition off part of the kitchen or perhaps an associated conservatory; somewhere where they can conveniently keep an eye on the litter and which, in turn, affords the puppies an opportunity to become accustomed to routine sights, smells, noise and so on typical of the normal household environment in which they are ultimately likely to live.

Suitable puppy pens are available to purchase or you can construct something similar utilizing wooden or part mesh panelling. Ideally these panels will hook or clip together so you can provide access for the bitch periodically. In this way extra panels can also be added later, as necessary, to provide a larger area as the litter gets older and the puppies require more room.

By three weeks of age the puppies' eyes will be open and, whilst their vision will be poor, they will start to hear what is going on around them. The fear response is not fully developed however in puppies of this age so it is the ideal time to start to introduce them to the sights and sounds of family life; sounds such as doorbells, the radio and television, doors opening and closing, and vacuum cleaners being used in the room but away from their pen.

You can buy CDs with these sounds on them or you can download them from the internet. They don't need to be played continuously but to be most beneficial, let the puppies hear these noises unexpectedly during the day at some time when they are awake. You don't need to play the sounds at full volume; what you are intending is for the puppies to notice the sounds and then quickly return to normal.

Anything your puppies see or hear now will be accepted as ordinary, notwithstanding the fact that they will startle on hearing unexpected sounds or when they appreciate sudden, unexpected movements. Such mild aversive stimulation will soon be forgotten at this age and their behaviour will quickly return to normal. This is how the litter will start to learn how to respond to non-threatening events as they further mature into adult dogs and in this way tend not to show the type of escalating fear response we associate with dogs that are 'gun shy', for example, or dogs that show any fear of strange people, other dogs or unusually loud noises such as fireworks.

At this age the puppy is also starting to learn about his social group. He learns to recognize his mother and his littermates, and to accept humans as being part of his extended family. This is a time when the bonding process begins.

Consequently this is an appropriate age at which to introduce other animals in the household, for example other fully vaccinated dogs and cats if you have them. Do not, however, introduce small animals such as rabbits, guinea pigs, hamsters and so on because you do not want to teach the puppies that these are part of their social group and that therefore it is acceptable to play with them; the hamster will certainly not enjoy it. Your puppies instead need to learn to ignore these animals.

Do all this quietly and gently; allow the other dogs to wander around outside the puppy pen, then pick up individual puppies so they can only smell and lick them initially without causing the puppy any undue concern. If they haven't been around already, this is also a good time to introduce children and other adults who you might want the puppies to appreciate as part of a wider family group.

It is generally far better to introduce novel items and expose puppies to unusual events and experiences too early than too late. A puppy's perception develops faster than its response, so they are often learning to appreciate – and most importantly cope with – mildly aversive stimuli and circumstances much sooner than we realize.

Worming

Start to regularly worm the litter once the puppies are three weeks of age. Worm treatment is simple and inexpensive. Regular worming is recommended not only to ensure no harm can come to the puppies but also for public health reasons; some types of worms commonly found in dogs can be passed on to humans.

Bitches should be wormed before breeding, during the last week of gestation, and each time the pups are wormed. Routine treatment of puppies and dogs, especially bitches, as well as environmental hygiene (picking up after your dog has passed faeces) are necessary and essential control measures.

Make sure any worming product that you use is not only effective but more importantly safe to use in puppies of this age and of their corresponding weight. You would be well advised to take advice from your vet on which worming product to use and on the most suitable way to administer the wormer. Some products for instance are sold in liquid form, suitable to dose with a syringe; others are available as tablets. You may find it much easier to dose puppies using a syringe or alternatively find it more reassuring knowing they have swallowed a tablet, and hence received the full dose, than risking one or two puppies regurgitating a liquid formulation and hence receiving only part of the dose.

The products that are currently most commonly used are as follows:

Fenbendazole is a broad-spectrum anthelmintic that can be used to both treat and control adult and immature roundworms. Fenbendazole is also effective in killing roundworm eggs. You should treat your puppies every two weeks with fenbendazole up to the point where they go to their new homes. Once they reach the age of twelve weeks they should thereafter be treated at three-monthly intervals. Fenbendazole is useful insofar as it is safe to use on very young puppies – as young as two weeks of age.

Combinations of **praziquantel, pyrantel embonate** and **febantel** have the advantage of being active against ascarids (roundworms, including both adult and late immature forms), hookworms, adult whipworms and tapeworms. Unfortunately it cannot be used to treat puppies less than 3kg bodyweight, but once they reach that size puppies can safely be treated every two weeks until twelve weeks of age and then at three-monthly intervals thereafter.

Using either of these products, it is not necessary to starve the puppies prior to worming as was often the case previously. Many older worming preparations tended to 'purge' the dog that then passed worms in its faeces. Don't be concerned if you don't see worms in the faeces after using most modern anthelmintics because the worms are killed high up in the gastrointestinal tract and processed naturally by digestive juices as they pass down the gut.

There now follows a brief description of the various types of worms that we commonly find in puppies, how they persist and the means of their control.

Roundworms

Dogs can harbour two types of large, ascarid roundworms (*Toxocara canis* and *Toxascaris leonina*). Although there are some species differences, for simplicity both species can be considered together. Both are found in the intestine of dogs and are a major public health concern because ascarid roundworms are transmissible to humans, especially children.

Prenatal infection occurs *in utero* when, influenced by the bitch's pregnancy, immature roundworm larvae migrate from her body tissues, muscles and other internal organs, to her uterus and thence infect the developing puppies via their placentae (the point where the pup attaches to the wall of the uterus via its umbilical cord). Most puppies are born with roundworms and early worming is an essential component of their control. Puppies can also become infected through the bitch's milk after larvae migrate to the lactating mammary glands.

Once within the puppy, the eggs hatch in the intestines. They then either develop directly into adult worms or migrate as larvae through the gut and into other tissues. Adult worms in the gut are about 60–70cm long and whitish in appearance, like pieces of string. Larvae in other tissues will remain dormant unless induced to migrate onwards to the intestine or, if it's a bitch, to the uterus during pregnancy. If the larvae migrate to the lungs, they will be coughed up and immediately swallowed to subsequently develop into adult worms in the intestine.

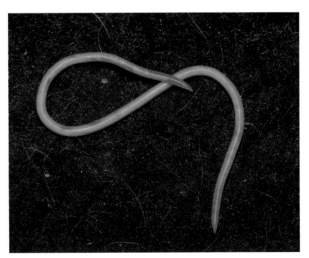

Depending on which anthelmintic (worming preparation) is used, you may see your puppies pass some adult worms that will look like small pieces of string, either in their stools or elsewhere in their pen.

Should the intestinal population be depleted, for instance by worming, then previously quiescent larvae will migrate to the intestine and replace those lost. This is why routine worming becomes so important.

It will therefore be obvious that roundworms have a complex life cycle to promote their survival and complicate roundworm treatment. The following are the essential points to note:

- Roundworms do not simply live in the gut. Their larvae survive in body tissues, for example the liver, lungs and skeletal muscle and remain there in a quiescent state.
- Roundworm larvae undertake active migration in pregnant bitches around the forty-second day of pregnancy.
- Roundworm larvae infect the foetal puppy via the umbilical vessels; initially they attack the pup's liver, then lungs at birth.
- Puppies can also become infected with roundworms through the bitch's milk when larvae migrate to lactating mammary tissues.

Tapeworms

Typically much longer than roundworms, a whole adult tapeworm is rarely seen as it is only segments of the adult worm body that are passed, as egg-carrying cases, in a dog's stools. The adult tapeworm comprises a small head that attaches by hooks arranged around its mouth to the wall of the dog's intestine, and a long body made up of numerous small individually discrete segments that are continuously formed at the head end of the parasite, and gradually maturate once they get further down the body of the worm. Once fully mature and full of eggs, these are constantly shed from the tail end of the tapeworm to be passed in the dog's faeces.

Tapeworms invariably use two hosts to complete their life cycle. An adult tapeworm in its definitive host, such as a dog, forms eggs that are shed to infect an intermediate host (a species that the definitive host will eat) where an infective form will develop awaiting consumption by the definitive host to form into an adult tapeworm and complete the cycle. *Dipylidium caninum*, the common dog tapeworm,

uses the flea as its intermediate host. If the puppy becomes infested with a tapeworm it will usually do so through coming into contact with fleas.

Tapeworm eggs can be seen in your dog's faeces or sticking to the hair around the dog's rear. These muscular segments of the worm are really egg cases, full of eggs and looking like a small, flattened grain of white rice that wiggle around spreading thousands of tapeworm eggs too small to be seen by the naked eye.

Lungworms

Lungworm infection in dogs, caused by the parasite *Angiostrongylus vasorum*, is becoming more prevalent in the UK. Dogs become infected through eating slugs and snails, which harbour the larvae of the parasite. Whilst most dogs do not habitually eat slugs and snails, they may often do so accidentally either when the slug or snail crawls on to a bone or toy left in the garden or from drinking from puddles and outdoor water bowls.

Lungworm can infect dogs of all ages, however younger dogs seem to be more prone to picking up the parasite and dogs having an active outdoor life, commonly visiting damp places, can be more at risk. With climate change bringing generally warmer, wetter winters, the parasite is now a nationwide threat.

A few simple precautions can help reduce the risk:

- Avoid the use of outdoor drinking water and food bowls. These tend to attract slugs and snails.
- Don't leave items like puppies' toys, chews and so on in places where they can attract snails.
- Ask your vet about recommending a parasite control programme that includes protection against lungworm infection, especially if you live in one of the higher risk areas.

Early feeding

At three weeks of age you can begin to introduce regular daily feeds so the puppies start to become accustomed to eating solid food. For this purpose you will need to feed the puppies away from the bitch and in this and other ways, allow the bitch increasingly long periods away from the puppies so they are not constantly drawing off milk and she can start to dry off. Feed the litter four or five times a day, depending on the type and size of the breed. Most breeds will be suitable for feeding four times daily, although others (primarily smaller dogs with correspondingly smaller appetites) will thrive better when fed five small meals.

Offer alternate 'meat' and 'milk' feeds through the day as previously described, so the puppy's digestive system has an opportunity to adapt gradually to the change from their bitch's milk to a diet made up almost entirely of 'solid' food.

FOUR TO FIVE WEEKS OF AGE

By four weeks of age the puppies should be starting to develop play behaviours, interact more energetically and, given the opportunity, beginning to develop problem-solving behaviour. This is a good time for them to start learning how to cope with the inevitable frustrations in life.

During this week, provide the litter with some early challenges; items to carry, pull, and climb upon. Add things that the puppies can begin to experiment with under your continuous supervision. Try introducing such items as Kongs, tunnels, upside-down cardboard boxes with holes cut out, or a handle-less bucket. Anything that is safe and under your supervision. Soft rope toys give the puppies something to move around and tug upon with their littermates. This all helps to develop strength, coordination, agility and sharing. Puppies deprived of such stimulation can grow up to be poor learners, unable to deal with frustration, which can result in serious behaviour or temperament problems later in life.

Don't be concerned if at this stage the bitch seems to be a little rough with her puppies at times; she might walk away when they are trying to suckle, or growl at them. It is important that you are not over-protective in these respects as she is teaching the puppies how to cope with and overcome some frustration.

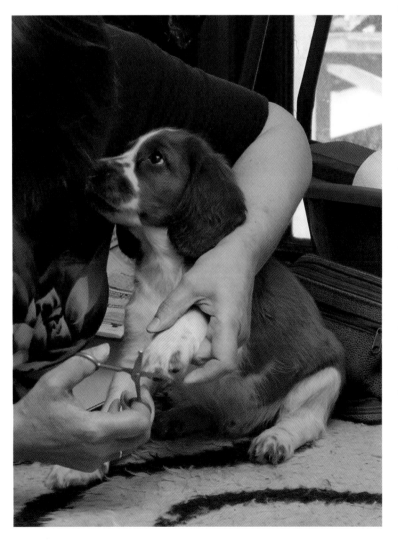

Puppies soon develop sharp toenails and it will usually be necessary to trim the tips with suitable nail clippers.

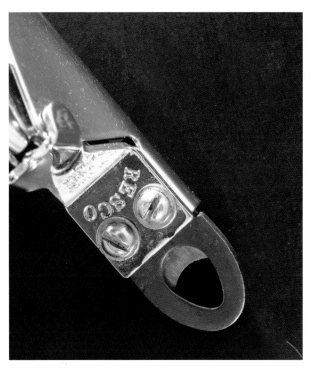

Guillotine-type nail clippers are popular. Close-up photograph of the clippers showing the guillotine blade.

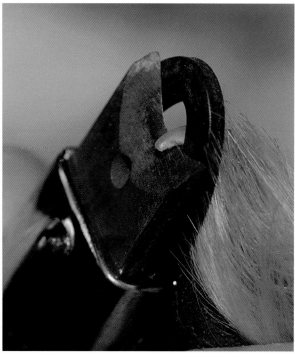

The tip of a toenail being clipped using guillotine nail clippers. Always hold the clippers with the guillotine blade on top, so you can see how much nail will be removed when making the cut.

This is the time to start spending more time with individual puppies. You can start to recognize their individual characteristics, traits and tendencies at this age and this will help later when you need to identify the most suitable homes for each of your puppies. Gradually increase the amount of time they spend away from their littermates and their mother. This will help to discourage them subsequently developing separation disorders and encourage their independence. It will also tend to reinforce their bonding with humans.

The sort of things to do once your puppies are around four to five weeks of age will include introducing them to different tactile experiences within the security of their puppy pen. They will, no doubt, have already experienced the feel of Vetbed or other similar soft bedding material so now is the time to start for example crunching up some of the newspaper in the pen. Try putting pieces of carpet, lino and/or rubber matting in the pen. Anything you can think of that would provide the puppies with lots of different tactile sensations, as long as the material is safe and the activity is under your constant supervision. Wherever possible provide them with a variety of tactile stimuli but avoid overwhelming the puppies.

Take each puppy out of the pen and spend a progressively longer time with him or her away from the littermates – up to ten minutes. During these periods continue getting the puppies used to being handled and having their mouths opened and their ears and feet examined. As soon as they are weaned onto solids you can start using tasty treats as a reward to ensure that being handled becomes associated with positive experiences.

Now is the time to teach each puppy to get used to being gently restrained. Kneel on the floor;

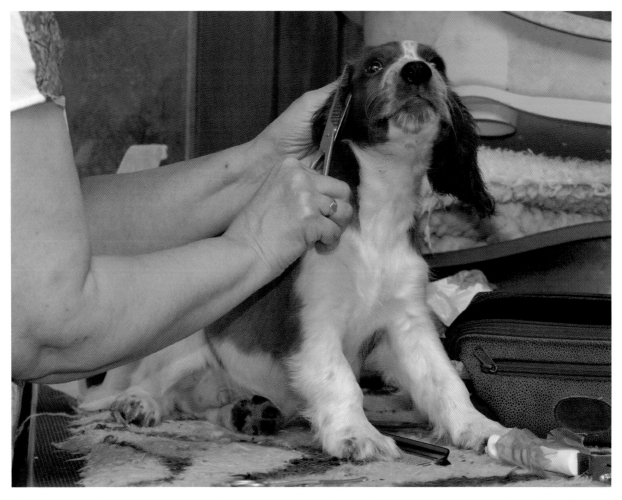

Grooming puppies from a young age is an extremely useful exercise. It not only separates them from their littermates but also teaches them to tolerate gentle restraint and, for those breeds that require regular grooming, makes the job significantly easier later in life.

hold a puppy between your legs with your hands linked across his chest. Restrain him like this gently for around three seconds provided he is calm and not wriggling. If the puppy starts struggling and resisting your restraint, don't fight him; better to give up and try again when he is more compliant. Always reward him for being good and in this way gradually increase the length of time so he gets used to dealing with the potential frustration of being restrained. Continue until such time as (later, when they are older) you can confidently restrain each of your puppies for a period of around thirty seconds.

By four to five weeks of age you can start to move the puppies as a litter around the house to different rooms with different noises, surfaces and activity levels. Start by allowing them to run around outside the pen whilst you clean it out. If the weather is favourable you can start carrying the litter out into the garden or onto the patio. This can provide an ideal opportunity to start house-training. As a general rule, puppies will tend to void urine and pass a motion immediately after being fed so take advantage of this tendency, take the puppies out immediately after each meal and wait until 'all is done'.

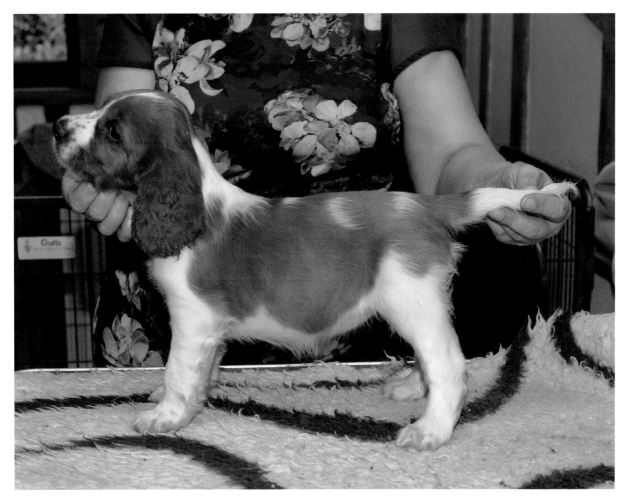

Get your puppies used to being gently restrained from an early age. This helps to ensure they are more manageable for their new owners, especially when having to be taken to the vet or otherwise restrained for training or treatment.

Reward good behaviour and then return each puppy to the pen. The litter will soon learn to associate meal times with this opportunity to go outside to relieve themselves, but always under supervision to avoid any accidents.

FIVE TO SEVEN WEEKS OF AGE

This is a critical period for the puppies in terms of their brain development. This is when they start to become curious about their immediate surroundings and the world beyond the puppy pen. They are willing to approach people, but at the same time their natural fearfulness starts to be shaped by their environment. Their fearfulness will start to gradually become more apparent over the next couple of weeks, so now is the time to introduce all manner of novel sights, sounds, people and other interesting experiences as this will all ultimately determine how well balanced the puppy will turn out as an adult.

Be aware of the fact that some breeds are more 'reactive' than others and in the more reactive breeds, the fear response and complementary hazard avoidance response starts earlier and increases more rapidly. In these breeds it is

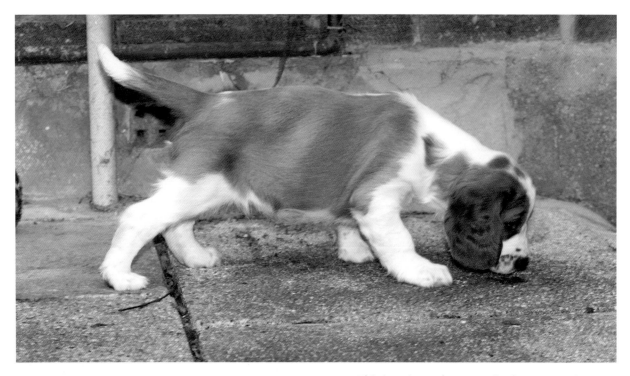

ABOVE: *This is a time when puppies become curious about their surroundings, so take the opportunity to allow them secure space outdoors if the weather permits so they can appreciate various novel experiences.*

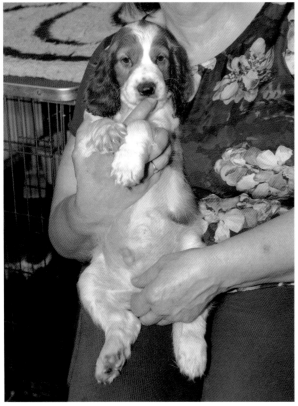

LEFT: *The manner of checking a male puppy to see if it has two testicles fully descended into the scrotum. Most will have descended by the age of twelve to sixteen weeks but some will descend earlier.*

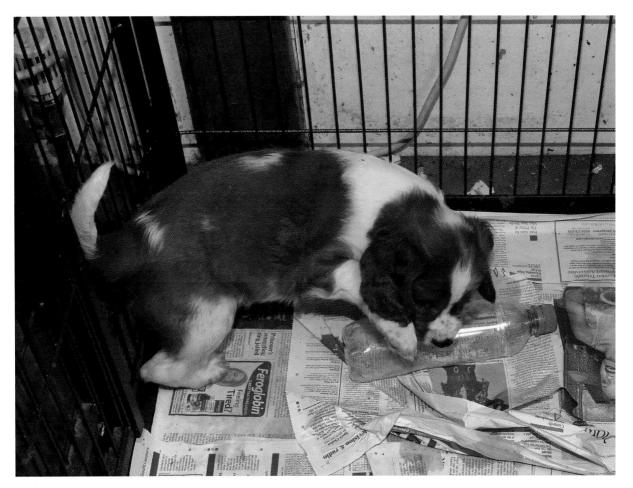

Something as simple as an empty plastic bottle can provide a puppy with various novel tactile and auditory sensations, plus hours of play and interaction with its littermates.

particularly important that the sort of activities described below are undertaken as early as possible at this stage of development whereas the less reactive, more stoical breeds have a later onset of hazard avoidance and so you can be a bit more relaxed when it comes to introducing these changes.

Hazard avoidance in the wild wolf (from which most domestic dogs are thought to be derived) starts around nineteen days of age. In the average dog it starts around forty-nine days old. For the German Shepherd Dog (one of the more reactive breeds) it starts around thirty-five days of age and in the Labrador Retriever (one of the

least reactive) it can start as late as seventy-two days of age. Note that these are all approximate dates as each dog is an individual and there will be some variation, nevertheless it serves to emphasize how important it is to work on these things through this particular two-week period.

This is also the time to begin teaching the puppies to start being left on their own away from their littermates, and to bond even more to humans. They are soon going to their new homes and getting used to being on their own at this stage will reduce the impact of leaving the litter and help them to settle in more quickly.

Suggested activities

1. Once the puppies are fully weaned and eating solid foods, start feeding them from different bowls. Introduce plastic and/or metal feeding bowls, and feed the puppies separately, away from their dam, and occasionally, if you can, individually away from littermates. Let them have their food a little bit away from you (perhaps in a crate, behind a chair). In this way the puppy will start to realize that good things can happen when he is on his own. Also on other occasions, feed them from your hand; they must learn that having humans around is always a good thing.

2. Introduce some more interactive toys into the puppy pen at times when you are around to supervise. This can include items like rolled-up pieces of carpet for the puppies to climb over, tunnel into or burrow under. Suspend balls from the top of the pen and/or provide larger Boomer balls that can be rolled about. Empty plastic bottles partly filled with pebbles will roll about making a noise when puppies play with them, cardboard boxes can be climbed on or in, and trays filled with stones or shallow water can be fun for them to play in... Anything you can think of that will represent novelty and positively stimulate your puppies.

3. Make sure the puppies meet as many different types of people as possible – both men and women, younger and older children, people with beards, people wearing hats, high-heel shoes, hoodies and so on. Make sure that these are each associated with some rewarding experience (treats or games for example).

4. With items like the TV and radio, vacuum cleaners, ironing boards and so on, always make sure that each of these new experiences is positive. Start very slowly with items that aren't moving or switched on, and reward the puppy with a treat for ignoring them and especially for not playing with them. Gradually you can work up to switching on the appliance, begin to move it around, at a distance at first and then getting closer. Always go back a step if the puppies react negatively and show any fear towards the item.

5. Spend time with the puppies, encouraging them to follow you, playing with them whilst making eye contact, stroking and handling them, picking them up and gently restraining them; generally getting them used to and enjoying human contact. Make sure all these interactions are positive for the puppies, always praise them and use treats as rewards if necessary.

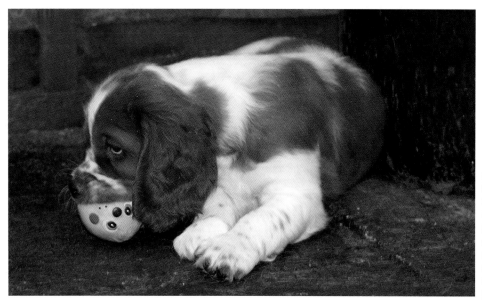

Balls come in various sizes, colours and materials. They make ideal toys for pups to play with but always make sure they are of a suitably safe material and always supervise young puppies' playtime.

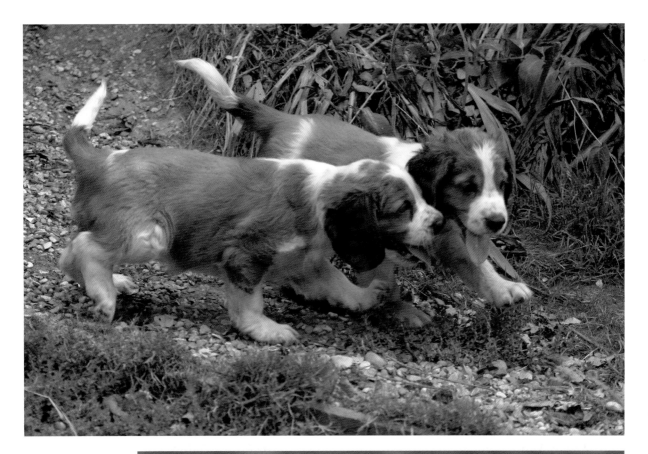

ABOVE AND RIGHT: *When the weather permits, allowing puppies to play (securely) outside is a useful opportunity for socialization. They will not only exercise and interact together, but also get used to exploring on their own, experience a whole range of tactile surfaces and learn to passively tolerate many background noises that might otherwise prove frightening when they are older.*

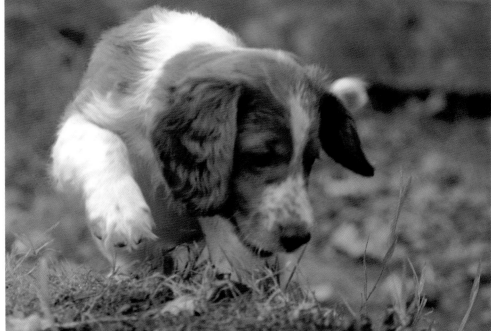

6. Take each puppy outside and sit it in the back of the car. As long as the puppy is relaxed and not alarmed by this new experience in a novel environment, start the engine. As soon as the puppy is used to the feel and sound of the engine, have someone help restrain the puppy, start to move off and drive round the block. He will soon start to see, hear and smell things that will be part of his future daily life (traffic for example). The litter will not be vaccinated yet (although they will still have some immunity passed on from the mother) so always carry the puppies out to the car, but this experience can be really important during these few weeks when their confidence is at its highest and their fear responses at their lowest.

7. Start getting the puppies used to wearing a light collar. Put the collars on for only a few minutes at first while they are preoccupied with doing other things. Do not leave collars on when they are unsupervised or in their playpen. The puppy will probably sit down and scratch the collar at first but they should gradually become accustomed to the feel of it and you can start to get them used to wearing one for longer periods of time.

The seven-week checklist

By the time the litter is seven weeks of age their early learning opportunities are nearly over and coming up to eight weeks of age you will be starting to think about getting ready to send them off to their new homes.

It is a good time to check that your puppies have experienced lots of different things and situations, meaning they will be less likely to be worried by unexpected situations or things that may happen in their new home.

By the time the litter is seven weeks old ideally they should have:

1. Met different types of people (such as babies, toddlers, children, women, men, people with walking sticks, umbrellas, hats, wheelchairs…).
2. Been on a variety of different surfaces (such as newspaper, carpet, lino, concrete, grass, polished floors, Vetbed, uneven ground…).
3. Played with different types of toys.
4. Heard different household/natural noises (for example TV, radio, vacuum cleaner, playing children, different traffic sounds, thunder, fireworks, things being dropped, cooking timers…).
5. Been in different locations (different rooms, or even different parts of the room), outside on concrete, on grass, hand-fed, in a car, with others, on their own and, ideally, been out and about to see different places or things (carried to watch traffic, children in playground, vets, sat in car and so on).

Think of including a list of these items in the 'puppy pack' that you provide for the new owners so they have a record of all the work that has been put into early training and socialization.

PREPARING PUPPIES FOR THEIR NEW HOMES

Provided you are well prepared, seek suitable advice and are responsible in mating your bitch and rearing her puppies, you should be rewarded with a fine litter that you will be proud to advertise and take great care in finding good homes

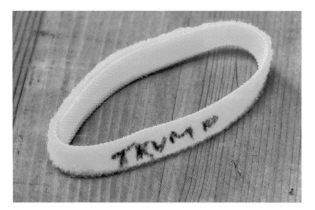

Small, light collars such as these, which are available in different colours, can also be useful to help you identify individual puppies.

for. It becomes all too easy to become attached to your puppies but by finding them suitable new puppy buyers, you can at least feel confident of their future well-being and anticipate hearing the satisfaction of their new owners.

Microchipping

A microchip is a tiny computer chip that's about the size of a grain of rice. It contains a unique code that matches up to your pet's details, which are recorded on a computerized database. Microchipping a dog is a quick and simple procedure.

As the breeder of the puppies, in the UK you must ensure that they are each microchipped and recorded on an authorized government-compliant database by the time they are eight weeks of age and before they go to their new homes.

Vaccination

You might choose to give the puppies a first vaccination prior to their going to new homes; your vet will be the best person to advise as he or she will be more aware of the disease risk in your area.

Vaccination consists of giving the dog a harmless dose of the infective agent, typically a virus or bacteria. The vaccine is typically rendered harmless either by first killing the agent, the standard method used to prepare bacterial vaccines, or by producing a so-called 'live' vaccine using a modified, non-infectious form of the disease-causing agent; this second method is often adopted when producing viral vaccines. When the dog is given a vaccine it will recognize it as something foreign and this induces an immediate immune response; the body creates what are known as antibodies against the agent in question. Antibodies will continue to be produced and circulate in the bloodstream, thereby recognizing and attaching to the infectious agent should the dog subsequently be exposed to the infection. The activated antibody attached to the infectious agent will then stimulate other parts of the dog's immune defence mechanism to fight and overcome infection.

There are essentially two means of producing a vaccine. 'Live' vaccines are intended to multi-ply once administered, mimicking infection and stimulating the immune response to produce antibodies. 'Killed' vaccines need to be administered on more than one occasion and usually as two doses given two to four weeks apart. The first dose of a killed vaccine will stimulate only a mild immune response but as soon as the second dose is given, the dog's immune system recognizes the vaccine and responds more vigorously, producing a much higher level of protection.

Puppies are normally given a first vaccination at six to eight weeks of age and a second at around twelve to fourteen weeks of age, although some vets in certain areas may advise delaying the final vaccination until the puppy is sixteen weeks of age. The apparent difference in advice between various veterinary practices is explained by problems arising from the variable persistence of maternal antibody protection – passive temporary protection that puppies receive from their dam through the 'first milk' when they start suckling immediately after birth. The bitch produces a substance called colostrum in the milk that transfers some of her immunity as antibodies.

Colostrum is only secreted by the bitch for twelve to thirty-six hours after whelping and it is obviously very important that puppies receive the benefit of this 'first milk'. The amount of protection provided for the puppy and the length of time over which it conveys protection depends entirely on how much colostral milk is consumed. Consequently individual puppies will vary in the amount of protection they receive from their mother and the period of time over which this protection lasts. The level of protection generally falls off between six to eight weeks of age but in many puppies, especially those that suckle vigorously after birth and receive most colostrum, it can persist until twelve to sixteen weeks of age. Maternal antibodies interfere with vaccination and if the level of maternal antibody remains high, there is risk that the vaccine won't 'take' and the puppy will be unprotected.

This obviously complicates matters since ideally the vaccine would be given as soon as the puppy's maternal antibody level declines to the

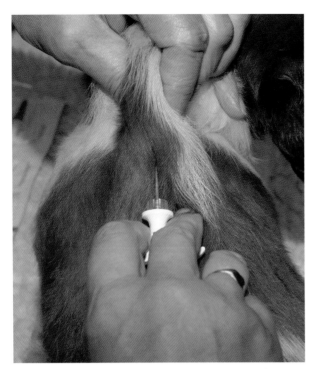

LEFT *The microchip is inserted under the dog's skin using a needle. It is usually inserted in the scruff of the neck, between the shoulder blades.*

BOTTOM: *Dogs can be checked for a microchip using a handheld electronic device called a scanner. When this is moved over the area where the microchip has been inserted, the scanner will recognize and display the unique information held inside the chip.*

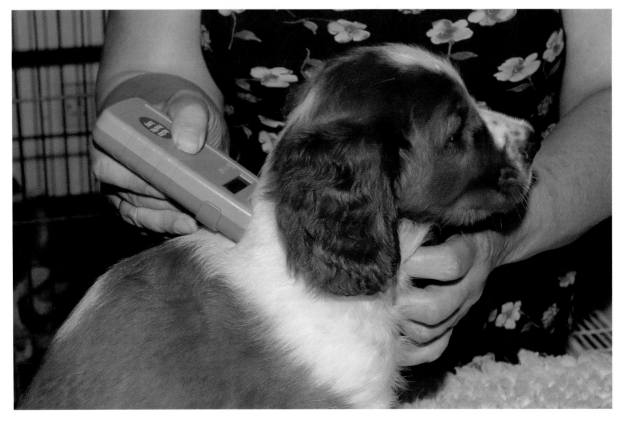

point where the vaccine can stimulate a strong immune response and induce the puppy to produce its own antibodies. Too soon and the vaccine won't take; too late and there is a risk that the puppy remains unprotected during the time after its maternal protection falls off until given the vaccine. The problem has been resolved to some extent by modern vaccines that are slightly more virulent and able to overcome low maternal antibody levels. It will be best to seek, trust and follow the advice of your veterinary surgeon. Your vet will not only understand the characteristics of the particular vaccines currently used in the practice but will also be aware of the relative disease risks in your particular area.

The diseases that are usually included in most multivalent canine vaccines include:

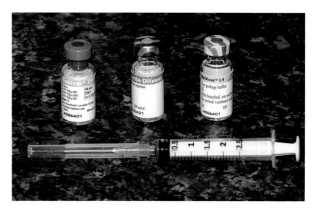

A typical canine vaccine comprises a vial containing a freeze-dried pellet (left), which prior to injection has to be dissolved in either the sterile water provided (centre) or mixed with another agent in liquid form. This example is a leptospirosis vaccine (right).

Canine distemper: A disease that affects dogs of all ages but is particularly common in puppies. It usually results in death and is characterized by respiratory signs such as runny eyes and nose, and nervous signs such as fits that may follow later.

Canine parvovirus: This is a distressing disease, often characterized by severe vomiting and profuse bloodstained diarrhoea that usually leads to dehydration and death. Again, it is common in puppies, but can affect and be fatal in older unvaccinated dogs.

Canine viral hepatitis: A very contagious disease. Symptoms include a high fever, jaundice, vomiting and stomach pains. Again, it can be fatal.

Leptospirosis: Dogs infected by the leptospira bacteria can suffer liver and kidney damage and require prolonged treatment if they are to fully recover.

Infectious bronchitis (kennel cough): Many of the more recent multivalent vaccines include viral antigens that help protect against infectious bronchitis, otherwise known as kennel cough. Kennel cough is frequently complicated by the presence of a bacterium called Bordetella bronchiseptica, which infects in addition to

these common viruses. The combined viral/bacterial infection causes respiratory disease ranging from a mild cough to severe bronchopneumonia. An intranasal vaccine provides protection against Bordetella bronchiseptica and is strongly recommended for dogs going anywhere where unfamiliar dogs congregate, such as working tests and field trials and especially into boarding kennels. Any boarding kennel should always ask to see your dog's certificate of vaccination before admitting the dog; if not, don't board your dog in the kennels!

Advise owners to take their vet's advice on how soon they are able to take their puppy out after vaccination to mix with other dogs. Until then they should be told not to exercise the puppy in places where other dogs are likely to have been. Your new owners will have a dilemma, ensuring that puppies are kept away from other dogs until fully vaccinated whilst at the same time ensuring that the puppy is well socialized whilst very young. Unfortunately there is no easy solution but experience shows that most puppies develop into well-socialized mature dogs despite the restrictions at this stage of development.

Preparing the new home
It might be helpful to provide the new owners with a list of items that they need to acquire in

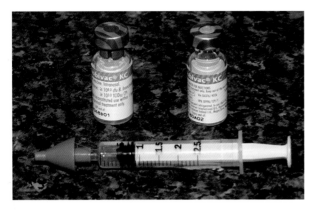

This intranasal vaccine provides protection against Bordetella bronchiseptica, *an important element of Kennel Cough infection. A special applicator is provided, attached to the syringe, to facilitate administrating the vaccine into the nostrils.*

advance of collecting their new puppy. The contents of the list will be somewhat dependent on the type of dog and the preferences of individual breeders but would likely include some or all of the following items:

- Puppy collar and lead.
- Feeding bowl and a separate bowl for drinking water.
- A suitable dog bed and/or a collapsible crate of your recommended type and size. A crate is useful in the first instance to help in transporting the puppy to its new home. If you recommend one, always make sure owners understand the correct use of the crate, as a refuge, and that it is not to be used to simply confine the dog.
- Suitable bedding. At least two pieces of suitable bedding material (so one is available whilst the other is being washed).
- Food. Make sure the new owners have a supply of the food that you have used to feed the puppies at the time they leave for their new homes. Advise the owners on where to acquire suitable food and the manner in which you feed both 'solid' and 'milk' feeds. This will help the puppy to settle in to its new home and minimize the likelihood of it developing a gut upset as it acclimates to any change in diet and water supply in the new environment.

Other useful equipment

It will be helpful to recommend that new owners acquire various products that contain dog appeasing pheromone (DAP). A DAP Adaptil diffuser could be set up near his cage to help him settle in; DAP can be sprayed on blankets both at home and on those used in the car when travelling, or a DAP collar (worn as well as his ordinary collar) will help calm the puppy when introducing him to new situations. It would be useful to have one ready on the day he goes to his new home.

Early training items, similar to any that you may have used already, would also be useful (a gundog whistle for example), as would advice on the precise type of product that you have been using, so the puppy recognizes it immediately.

Recommending suitable interactive toys that have proven to have more than mere novelty value can save your new owners wasted time and money buying items their new puppy plays with initially and then completely ignores. For example, he will enjoy retrieving a canvas puppy dummy for you when you are training and these are a good starting weight to pick up. Other puppies might like soft, disc-shaped toys to retrieve or ones that are half-covered in fur. Simple rope 'pullers' are often popular but make sure the new owner is aware of how to use them so they do not risk damage to developing jaws and teeth.

Routine treatment for parasites

Worm your puppies before they leave for their new homes and use a suitable flea spray as a prophylactic treatment for ectoparasites prior to departure.

Provide the new owners with the details of all treatments that you have provided for your puppies, including details of the product(s) used and the dates of the treatments so the owner can pass this information on to their veterinary surgeon when first registering their puppy. Their vet can then use this information when advising on further routine treatments.

The 'puppy pack'

Try to put together all the essential information, items appropriate for the puppy's immedi-

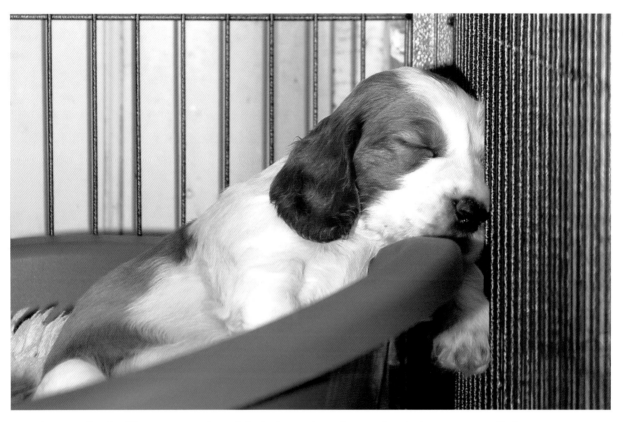

Puppies spend a significant proportion of their time asleep. Remember to impress upon their new owners the importance of allowing them time alone to rest.

ate care in its new home, and/or material that the new owners will find helpful as a 'puppy pack', ready to hand over when people collect their puppy. You will probably want to tailor the contents of your puppy packs according to individual circumstances and preferences but, for example, a typical pack might include:

- Your contact details as the breeder
- The pedigree form
- Kennel Club Registration document (if appropriate) together with –
- Copy of any agreement regarding endorsements you may have indicated on the Kennel Club registration, signed by new owner and breeder
- Insurance cover note
- Microchip details, with instructions on how to record the change of ownership

- Vaccination certificate
- Puppy sales contract
- Puppy advice notes (*see* below)
- Copies of relevant health test results for the puppy's sire and dam
- Details of grooming equipment and where to buy (new owner already been shown how to groom, clean ears, trim nails prior to taking puppy)
- Piece of familiar bedding
- Next meal – mixed and ready to feed.

Written notes for new owners

Even though you may spend a lot of time explaining to new owners how to first feed, house-train and generally look after their new puppy, it is always helpful to provide suitable notes for them to refer to subsequently. At the time of collecting their new puppy, people will naturally be more

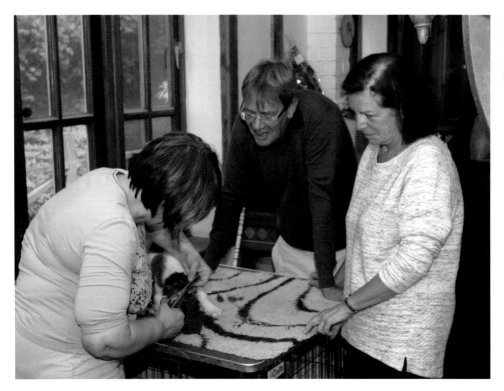

It is often helpful if you demonstrate to novice owners how to trim excess hair, give routine treatments, etc.

focussed on the puppy itself and their plans for taking it away and settling it in to their home environment than really concentrating on all that you are telling them.

Useful information to provide in this context might include details of:

- Vaccination
- Worming
- Flea and any other ectoparasitical treatment
- Nutrition; what you recommend feeding, when and how to feed it, and how to reduce the number of daily feeds as their puppy gets older
- House-training
- Insurance
- Exercise
- Socialization and training.

It may also be appropriate to outline any breed-related traits and tendencies and/or to recommend any books on the breed or other information, such as on the internet, that they may find useful. Some owners may be interested in becoming more involved with their dog and would appreciate details of the relevant breed clubs, training classes and so on in their area.

You will no doubt have established a rapport with your new owners during the occasions when they have made preliminary enquiries about a suitable puppy, visited to see your puppies and finally spoken with you on the day they collect their new puppy. They will normally require further help over the first few days and weeks, especially whilst the puppy is first settling in. Expect them to turn to you for help in the first instance and be prepared to offer further advice.

6 THE USE OF ARTIFICIAL INSEMINATION

Artificial insemination means the intentional implantation of sperm into a female's reproductive tract for the purpose of achieving a pregnancy by means other than sexual intercourse. The technique is regularly used as a fertility treatment for humans, and has become common practice for animal breeding, especially in the breeding of dairy cattle, horses and pigs. Artificial insemination will normally employ assisted reproductive technology that will involve semen collection, evaluation and preservation, and various particular animal husbandry techniques.

Dog breeders are finding artificial insemination (AI) to be a valuable tool and a viable alternative

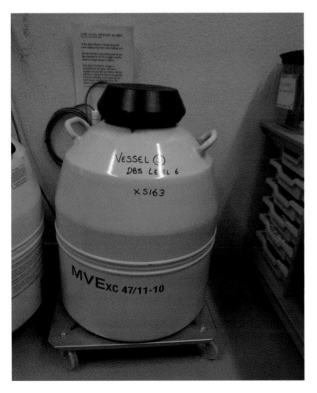

to natural mating, primarily because it enables them to use semen from dogs that might not otherwise contribute to the gene pool in their kennel. These days the actual technique and methods of artificial insemination are relatively simple and can be accessed by UK dog breeders relatively easily as the service is now offered by a number of private individuals and particular specialist veterinary clinics.

Although the use of artificial insemination is still relatively new in canine medicine, it has been successfully practised in cattle and other species for many decades. Unfortunately, although the canine AI technologies are based on much of the research undertaken and the experience gained in developing the use of artificial insemination in cattle, we have yet to duplicate the high rate of success achieved in bovine and porcine practice. This is not because the technique in dogs is in any way inferior, but reflects the relative instability of canine sperm when it is either frozen or chilled, compared to that from pigs and cattle. In addition, we have to understand that cattle and pigs have been consistently selected for reproductive efficiency whereas this is not the case in dogs. Compared to dogs, pigs and cattle have more predictable oestrus cycles and are selected partly on the basis of their fertility and fecundity. Dog breeders are generally more

Stored in liquid nitrogen at -196°C in special storage vessels such as this, frozen semen has been successfully preserved for many decades.

emotionally attached to their animals and select them on the basis of other criteria; even repeatedly attempting to breed from 'problem' bitches (in the reproductive sense) and breeding from bitches with irregular cycles. All this is in distinct contrast to the situation that currently prevails in the commercial pig and dairy industries.

Nevertheless, provided the bitch is properly inseminated and accepting that the success rate can vary with the skill of the inseminator, the success rates achieved with artificial insemination can mirror those achieved through natural breeding. Using semen that is fresh and has been chilled, the success rate can be as high as 80 per cent and whilst frozen semen placed directly into the vagina is associated with a relatively low success rate, transcervical insemination of frozen semen (depositing it directly into the uterus via the cervix) has, on average, a success rate of around 60–80 per cent. In general terms the success rate in achieving canine pregnancies using AI is largely dependent on three factors: the quality of the semen being inseminated, the accurate timing of when to inseminate, and the site of deposition of the semen.

THE ADVANTAGES OF ARTIFICIAL INSEMINATION

Geographical and temporal AI

This offers a means of overcoming the limitations of both distance and time. Frozen semen from dogs can be stored and kept for many years, certainly decades, and enables breeders to potentially choose to use virtually any dog in the world. Consequently, an exceptional male, chosen for his conformation, performance, intelligence and personality can continue to produce offspring long after his death, or be mated with females from which he is separated by thousands of miles.

Reproductive efficiency

One ejaculate can be split into multiple semen doses for AI. Those doses can then be used for repeated breeding to one bitch, or to breed with many bitches. By preserving and storing his semen, a stud dog will be able to breed with many

more females than would be physically possible through normal one-on-one natural mating.

Similarly, by inseminating a bitch with mixed semen from two stud dogs there is a very good chance that offspring in the resulting litter will represent the progeny of both sires. Provided the dam and her sires are each DNA profiled, individual littermates can be genetically tested, their sire identified and then registered accordingly with their true parentage and be available to contribute in future to the gene pool in the breed.

Overcoming physical handicaps

There have been cases where valuable stud dogs have been injured and can no longer mount a female. Despite their injury, their genetics are unaltered, and artificial insemination allows them to continue to contribute to their breed.

Forward planning

A mating with a promising young bitch that has the potential to improve a kennel through her progeny can be planned even though the appropriate stud dog may be retired or deceased by the time she is in heat and ready to be mated. Through the use of AI, plans can be made to collect, freeze and store the stud dog's semen, until such time as she is of a suitable age and ready to be bred.

Convenience and welfare

For owners using chilled or frozen semen, AI allows them to breed from their dogs whenever it is convenient. Shipping semen is much more convenient (and quite often cheaper) than transporting a bitch to be mated and offers certain advantages in terms of the animal's welfare. No matter how accustomed a dog is to travelling, taking a male outside of his normal environment can cause insecurity and make his attention wander and a consequential long journey for a bitch in heat can increase her stress levels. Similarly for both dogs, transportation will also incur some increased, albeit minor, risk of accidental injury. Alternatively, frozen semen can be shipped in advance and stored locally in preparation for the bitch to be inseminated when the time is right.

Expanding the gene pool and enhancing genetics

A small gene pool and limited genetic diversity can cause reduced biological fitness and carries an increased risk of extinction. A small gene pool also enables genetic disease to be passed on more easily since there is greater opportunity for two dogs with the same genetic disease being mated together. Artificial insemination extends the choice of stud males to those available overseas and this makes it possible for breeders to genetically diversify their dogs.

Reduced risk of sexually transmitted disease and infection

Because there is no physical contact through AI, the technique prevents both dogs from passing on or contracting sexually transmitted diseases, such as canine transmissible venereal tumours, brucellosis and canine herpes virus; diseases that can cause cancer, abortion, or sterility. AI also helps prevent infection occurring following any injury incurred during mating. There is, however, a risk from certain diseases that can be transmitted through infected semen and consequently prior blood testing of donor animals as well as semen evaluation is usually required prior to semen collection and insemination, respectively.

SEMEN COLLECTION

Most male dogs will allow semen to be collected. Normally a stud dog is easily aroused when presented with a bitch in oestrus (although with some stud dogs this is not always necessary) and once the male dog adjusts to being assisted, the semen can easily be collected.

Typically, to collect semen the male dog is first introduced to the in-season female and, once excited, will attempt to mount her. Before the male can insert his penis into her vagina, however, it is grasped and deflected to one side, into an artificial vagina or other suitable receptacle in which to collect the semen. An artificial vagina comprises a cylindrical rubber jacket filled with warm water at 37°C to one end of which is attached the actual collection receptacle. Whatever form of receptacle is used, it should ideally be

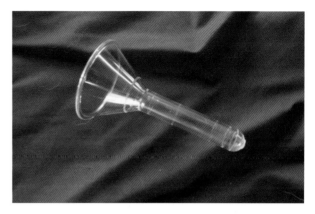

A special plastic, single-use, disposable collection funnel for collecting semen.

made of glass and warmed to body temperature prior to collection because sperm are extremely susceptible to cold shock and some types of rubber and plastic can be spermicidal.

By continually massaging the penis to simulate the constriction of the vagina during normal breeding, ejaculation will be achieved and semen can be collected. If a collection vessel or funnel is used, semen should not be collected until full erection is achieved and thrusting movements have ceased so as not to damage the penis.

The ejaculate comprises three distinct fractions. The first and last fractions consist of prostatic fluid which accounts for about 95 per cent of the total volume ejaculated. Prostatic fluid is believed to assist the successful deposition of semen by flushing the female reproductive tract whilst the dogs are tied during mating. The second (intermediate) fraction is sperm-rich and if the semen is to be frozen and stored, only this second sperm-rich fraction is normally collected. Alternatively, prostatic fluid can be collected in the receptacle if the semen is to be used immediately. Semen can be collected twice at thirty-minute intervals from most dogs.

Once semen has been collected, the male's penis can be withdrawn from the artificial vagina or otherwise removed from the collection receptacle, being careful not to cause any damage to the engorged penis. The stud male is then nor-

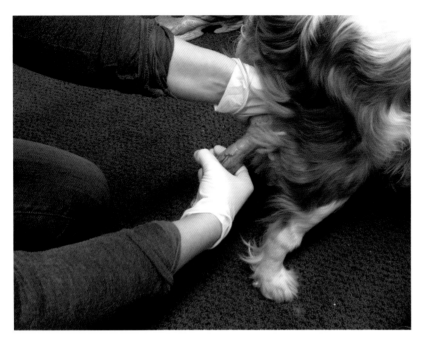

Collecting semen from a dog. Note how the engorged penis is being directed backwards in the same way as it is when the dog is 'tied' to the bitch during natural mating.

In assessing semen quality it is customary to evaluate the following characteristics.

Gross appearance

The sperm-rich fraction of the ejaculate will normally be white and creamy. A yellowish tinge is likely to indicate that the sample is contaminated with urine. A yellow or green colour might indicate the presence of inflammatory cells or pus, thereby indicating some form of infection, and the presence of blood in the ejaculate would impart a reddish or brown tinge. If the ejaculate were to appear clear or cloudy with no change in its colour, the sperm density in the sample is likely to be low or there may even be no spermatozoa present at all in the semen and the dog is likely to be sterile.

mally removed from the room to avoid any further attempts to mount the female.

If a bitch in heat is unavailable, breeders will often keep a supply of cotton swabs that have been wiped across an oestrus bitch's vaginal area and stored in a refrigerator. Such swabs can then be wiped across the vaginal area and over the back of another female dog so that the male will smell the pheromones produced by the oestrus female and think that the bitch is in season.

SEMEN ASSESSMENT

Following collection, semen should always be properly evaluated prior to its use for immediate insemination and/or preservation by either chilling or freezing. This is primarily to assess its likely potential to be fertile and to ensure that there are no obvious abnormalities or anomalies that might adversely influence the outcome of either insemination or preservation.

Volume

Typically this will be measured immediately after collection in a graduated test tube. The first fraction of a dog's ejaculate will normally be around 0.5–2.0ml. The second (sperm-rich) fraction will be around 0.5–3.0ml and there will be 5 to 20ml of the third (prostatic) fraction. These volumes are largely dependent on the size of the dog.

Motility

Sperm motility is assessed microscopically. A drop of semen is placed on a microscope slide and examined under the microscope. Sperm motility is highly influenced by temperature so it is customary to use a slide warmed to body temperature and ideally the microscope will be equipped with a heated 'stage' on which the microscopy slide is placed whilst the semen is being examined. The degree of motility will be subjectively scored and expressed as a percentage of the sperm seen actively progressing across the field of view under the microscope. Motility may also be categorized, where 0 indicates non-motile spermatozoa (which will be infertile) through incremental steps up to 5, which implies that the semen comprises rapidly progressive spermatozoa. Good-quality semen will have at least 70 per cent of the sperm categorized as 5.

Microscopic appearance

Also referred to as morphology. A number of sperm in the sample, typically around 100–200, will be examined under a high-power microscope and the appearance of any abnormal sperm in that sample will be noted. A spermatozoa comprises a head, midpiece and tail and if any defects or anomalies are detected in any of the constituent parts of any individual sperm, these will be noted. Some of the defects that are commonly seen are related to the age/maturity of the sperm and might reflect, for instance, prolonged sexual rest. Others have more serious implications; sperm with coiled tails are unlikely to be capable of progressing up the uterus to reach the oviducts to fertilize an egg. Defects detected in the midpiece are usually associated with infertility in dogs.

Semen quality can vary with time, in particular the age of the dog and the time of year when the sample is collected. The dog's ancestors were, and their surviving relatives remain, seasonal breeders. This seasonality has been largely bred out of domestic dogs, especially bitches, but males tend to have a much higher sperm count in the spring and it tends to decline during the summer. For obvious reasons it makes sense to avoid collecting and storing semen during periods when the quality might be adversely affected.

There is no proven correlation between the percentage of abnormal sperm and fertility. Nevertheless, our observations and experience indicate that semen should be considered to be of acceptable quality if it contains at least 80 per cent normal, motile sperm. Samples with a significantly lower percentage are likely to be considered unsuitable. This is particularly important if the semen is to be frozen because not only is there a risk of the dog being sterile, but an unacceptably low percentage of his sperm are likely to survive the freezing process and therefore it will be incapable of subsequently fertilizing a bitch.

It is important to understand that the assessment described here is of semen quality and that this does not necessarily reflect a dog's fertility. A dog with low-quality sperm might still be fertile and able to successfully achieve a pregnancy. To properly assess fertility we have to try breeding from the dog to be assured that he is capable of achieving successful pregnancies among the bitches that he inseminates.

SEMEN STORAGE

Interest in using artificial insemination for the breeding of dogs has increased significantly over the past four decades. Unless the semen is to be collected and transferred directly into a recipient bitch, there are two primary means of preserving semen prior to its subsequent insemination. It may be diluted, cooled ('chilled') and stored at 5°C for several days and then used for insemination, or the semen may be diluted ('extended') in a suitable cryoprotectant solution and stored under liquid nitrogen at -196°C.

Cryopreservation of canine semen like that of other animal species is used for artificial insemination and for the long-term storage of semen samples from valuable stud dogs. Frozen semen can be stored and kept for many years, even decades, and enables dog breeders to breed their bitches with virtually any dog in the world and/or with valuable dogs that are long deceased. Since the first birth of live offspring from frozen dog semen was recorded in 1969, the cryopreservation of dog semen has become particularly popular because it allows the shipment of semen and thereby the transfer of valued genetic material both within and between countries, even those separated by many thousands of miles.

In developing these new techniques for semen preservation, the goal has been to minimize any damage caused to the spermatozoa by the chilling or freezing process(es) in order to recover the maximum number of viable sperm after its storage.

Irrespective of the process used, cryopreservation results in reduced fertility compared to natural mating using fresh semen. This situation arises from a combination of factors: reduced sperm viability as well as some impaired function of those sperm that survive the freezing and storage processes. This needs to be borne in mind whenever breeding strategies involving AI are being contemplated. We need to develop and use cryopreservation processes that not only optimize the proportion of sperm surviving after freezing, but also the capability of those surviving sperm to successfully achieve pregnancy in any bitches inseminated with the stored semen.

CHILLED SEMEN

Fresh-chilled semen refers to semen that is collected, cooled and shipped immediately to inseminate a bitch that is at peak ovulation, or going to ovulate while the semen is in transit.

Chilled semen can survive and fertilize eggs for around five days after collection as long as it is kept at the correct temperature. However, it normally needs to be shipped to a bitch and the conditions of shipment impose certain additional time constraints. Generally the special chilled semen transport boxes that are available will keep the semen at the correct temperature for about forty-eight hours. Consequently, organizing the collection and shipment to coincide with an ideal insemination time for the bitch is essential. Chilled semen can be sent to a breeder in another area of the UK or Europe or even, in certain cases, to North America if there are appropriate flights and courier services available to enable the journey to be made within the requisite forty-eight-hour period.

Chilled semen once inseminated doesn't survive as long as fresh semen so progesterone testing of the bitch is necessary to estimate the best time to collect the semen and to know exactly when to inseminate.

It is recommended that the semen is evaluated both before cooling to ensure that the sample quality is good enough to use chilled and, ideally, again after chilling to ensure it remains suitable for insemination prior to packing and shipping.

Packaging fresh-chilled semen

Preparation for shipping is an important step in the process of using fresh-chilled semen. Great care must be taken to prepare the semen properly and to package and ship it correctly. A typical container suitable for packaging and shipping chilled semen includes:

- An insulated Styrofoam container
- Solid-frozen gel-ice packs
- Tube(s) to contain the extended (diluted) semen sample(s)
- A sturdy cardboard box that fits snugly around the insulated container.

The method of shipping is also critical. Packages that are shipped in a non-pressurized compartment of an aircraft will cause the sample to become frozen, and rendered useless for breeding. Care must be taken therefore to label the package as a biological sample that must be placed in a pressurized area of the aircraft.

Transporting chilled semen is much cheaper than transporting frozen semen, but the downside of using chilled semen is having to coordinate collection, transport and insemination.

Insemination

Chilled semen can be inseminated into the anterior vagina but best results are achieved if the semen is deposited in the uterus using a transcervical insemination technique.

FROZEN SEMEN

Canine semen can be successfully frozen and subsequently thawed and used to inseminate bitches in almost any country in the world, and at any time in the future. Puppies have already been produced from semen that has been frozen for over thirty years.

Some breeds of dogs in the UK have a limited gene pool and using a stud from another country may help to maintain and improve the genetic health of the breed. Using semen from a stud dog frozen many years previously also enables breeders to reintroduce genetic material and physical characteristics that may subse-

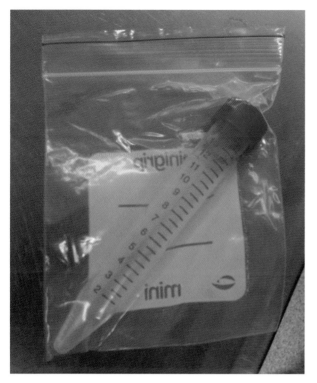

A sample of semen (within the red-topped tube) packaged ready for chilling and shipping. The sample tube should be securely sealed within a plastic bag to prevent any loss of semen should the tube accidentally leak during shipment.

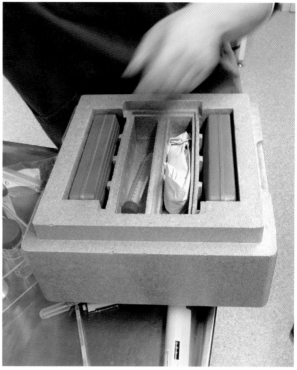

A consignment of chilled semen ready for shipping. Two (blue) ice packs within the insulated container help keep the semen chilled whilst in transit.

quently have become limited or lost from a previous breeding line. Freezing a stud dog's semen while he is young can represent an insurance and enables him to continue to produce puppies even if he later becomes infertile or suffers severe injury. It also, of course, enables his genetic potential to be used for future generations of puppies.

The freezing process and the transport of frozen semen are more expensive than the equivalent preservation and transport costs of chilled semen. However, it does allow for collection at a time that is optimal and/or convenient and the semen can then be shipped and ready for use well in advance of the date it is required for insemination. It means that we normally avoid freezing semen during the summer months when semen quality is generally poorer and do not need to coordinate semen collection with the time of ovulation.

The freezing and thawing processes do fundamentally influence the motility and subsequent fertilizing potential of the sperm, so only good-quality semen samples should be stored. The success of using frozen semen is also highly dependent on the method of insemination, meaning that it needs to be deposited directly into the uterus.

Preparation and storage of frozen semen

Since semen quality is more critical when it comes to freezing, each semen sample needs to be evaluated prior to starting the process. As part of the collection and preparation process, prostatic fluid is removed and the sperm-rich fraction to be used must be diluted with a suitable

ADVANTAGES OF SEMEN CHILLING IN COMPARISON WITH CRYOPRESERVATION

- Less spermatozoa are damaged during chilling than after freezing-thawing
- Lower transport costs
- Cheaper cost per dose
- Good results can be achieved by depositing semen into the vagina. This method does not require either special techniques or sedation and can be easily repeated.

DISADVANTAGES OF SEMEN CHILLING IN COMPARISON WITH CRYOPRESERVATION

- Chilled semen cannot be stored for a long time
- Immediate transport at a constant temperature of 5°C and subsequent immediate insemination are necessary.

cryoprotectant (which we usually refer to as an extender). Semen is normally titrated to a laboratory standard as it is diluted, so that when subsequently used for insemination the number of live, motile sperm in the sample is known.

The sample is then cooled to 5°C before being transferred for freezing and storage in 0.5ml plastic straws. These straws are individually identified, normally with the name of the dog, its Kennel Club registration and/or microchip number, the date of freezing and the name of the laboratory/clinic that collected and processed the semen.

The straws filled with extended semen are then frozen using either a manual or automated process, and then stored in large flasks of liquid nitrogen at -196°C. After freezing a test straw will be thawed and the motility of the sperm cells will be checked. It is the number of live, motile sperm after thawing that determines how many straws are needed for future inseminations.

As an alternative, the extended semen can be stored as pellets after cooling. For this purpose it is pipetted directly onto blocks of frozen carbon dioxide (dry ice) and the resulting solid drops of semen are collected and transferred to small plastic cryotubes, with each tube containing sufficient pellets to constitute a breeding dose.

Normally the straws or pellets that are frozen remain the immediate property of the stud dog owner at the time of collection. Frozen semen can remain viable for many years, certainly many decades, and has been known to survive longer than its immediate owner. Consequently, to enable its continued use and for any progeny to be registered with the Kennel Club, it is advisable to make suitable arrangements regarding future ownership.

Transportation

Frozen straws are transported in a 'dry shipper', which has liquid nitrogen absorbed into it. This means it is safe to transport and the straws inside should remain frozen for several days. These dry shippers are expensive to purchase and need to be returned to the clinic. They need to be 'charged' prior to use, which involves slowly cooling the interior of the shipper using liquid nitrogen so that the container remains at the required (very low) temperature for the necessary period during which the sample is to be shipped. Dry shippers are also quite heavy and so transport costs are not insignificant, however with prior knowledge it is possible to share costs with another owner exporting straws to the same destination. More recently, a 'disposable' shipper, often called a 'cryodrum', has become available. It is lighter and does not need to be returned to the clinic. Unfortunately it keeps the straws at -196°C for a shorter period of time and so may not always be

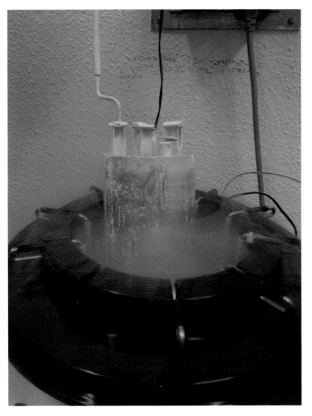

These 'canes' being withdrawn from the storage vessel are used to hold straws containing the cryopreserved semen under liquid nitrogen. The canes can be conveniently labelled, enabling sample straws from individual dogs to easily be identified and withdrawn from storage when required for subsequent insemination.

An individual cane withdrawn to show how straws containing frozen semen (arrowed) are held in plastic 'goblets' that clip on to the cane. In this system each cane holds two goblets, each containing up to ten straws, four to five straws being typically used for each insemination.

suitable for international shipments where journey times may be longer.

International shipments

Depending on the country of destination, the stud dog may have to undergo certain health tests prior to collecting and sending the semen. The high health status of dogs in the UK means this is often not required but it is advisable to check with the Animal Health and Plant Agency (AHPA) in Carlisle and with the corresponding authority in the country of destination prior to the bitch coming into season.

To import chilled semen into the UK, the stud must have a valid PETS passport. An import licence is also necessary and in certain cases an export licence from the country of origin may be required.

INSEMINATION

The success of using artificial insemination in the breeding of dogs is highly dependent on a number of critical factors:

- Using semen of appropriate (high) quality
- Using an appropriate technique for insemination, depending on the type of semen being used
- Timing insemination so that it closely corresponds with the time of ovulation.

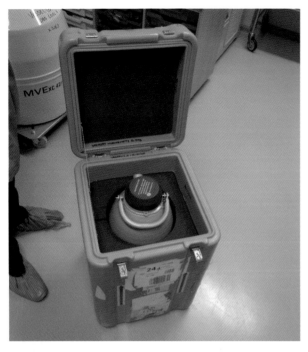

A dry shipper within a special transport container used to keep it secure during transit. Frozen canine semen can be safely transported for periods of up to five days in such shippers.

The timing of insemination

Unfortunately there is no sure way of detecting when a bitch's ova (eggs) are ready to be fertilized. We can only estimate the best time by considering what happens in the average bitch and then allow for variation. Bitches normally ovulate twelve to forty-eight hours after first accepting the male but the ovulated eggs are immature at this stage and require a further twenty-four to forty-eight hours to maturate before they can be fertilized. The mature ova can probably survive for a further twenty-four to thirty-six hours before dying.

Some bitches may ovulate before showing oestrus (the time during which they will accept the male) and others may not ovulate until much later. Consequently, it is useful to measure when ovulation occurs. This can be done by monitoring hormone levels, as previously described in Chapter 2, and the measurement of circulating progesterone concentration is considered a reliable tool to determine the optimum time for insemination using AI.

Whether to use one or two inseminations will largely depend on how accurately ovulation can be detected and on the quality of the semen being used. When fresh or chilled semen is used it is customary to inseminate on the day of ovulation and again two days later. When using frozen semen however, we have to bear in mind the fact that its longevity is reduced by the freezing and thawing processes. Because canine oocytes (eggs) must mature in the oviduct after ovulation and prior to fertilization, insemination is normally delayed until two days after ovulation and, ideally, a second insemination may be carried out two days later.

There is some discrepancy within the literature concerning the range of progesterone concentration at ovulation. Most inseminators, however, will have prior experience and can advise on an optimum range to determine when to inseminate that has proven successful in association with the particular technique that they use. Always heed this advice and follow any instructions provided by the clinic you have chosen to carry out the insemination.

By way of illustration, in one clinic the following criteria are recommended:

- Progesterone concentration of 15–24nmol/l (5–8ng/ml): perform the first AI two days later and repeat after twenty-four hours
- Progesterone concentration of 25–34nmol/l (8–11ng/ml): inseminate immediately and repeat two days later
- Progesterone concentration of 35–60nmol/l (11–20ng/ml): inseminate immediately and repeat one day later
- Progesterone concentration of >60nmol/l (20ng/ml): inseminate immediately as ovulation has already occurred.

Thawing semen

The required number of straws containing frozen semen are taken from the liquid nitrogen and immersed directly into a water bath at 37 to 40°C for one minute. The straws are then dried, the sealed end cut off with scissors and the semen expelled into a sterile plastic tube without further dilution. Alternatively the semen may be expelled into a tube containing similarly warmed thawing solution prior to insemination.

Frozen semen in pellets can be thawed by direct immersion into a pre-warmed solution at 37 to 40°C. Pellets are removed from the cryo-tube with forceps under liquid nitrogen and then dropped immediately into the thawing medium held in a sterile plastic tube. Once all the pellets have been transferred, the tube is vigorously swirled for thirty seconds; the thawed semen can then be evaluated and used for insemination as appropriate.

When frozen semen is thawed, its motility will initially be quite slow but will usually pick up rapidly when examined under a microscope on a slide that has been pre-warmed to 37 to 40°C. Post-thaw motility of good-quality semen will be in the order of 50–70 per cent or higher. Motility may vary depending on the extender that was used but there will normally be no more than a 20 per cent loss of motility compared to that observed in the fresh semen sample prior to freezing.

INSEMINATION TECHNIQUES

Whilst performing AI, semen may be deposited either in the vagina or directly into the uterus. There are two principal ways of depositing semen into the uterus; it may either be introduced through the cervix and into the uterus (a technique described as transcervical insemination) or it may be deposited directly into the uterus by surgically (laproscopically) inserting an AI device into the uterus which obviously will require an operation performed under general anaesthesia. Each has advantages and disadvantages and all are more (or less) suitable depending on the technique employed to achieve insemination.

Vaginal insemination

This is relatively simple to perform and may be carried out using a plastic catheter, to which a syringe can be attached, or a pipette. Suitable catheters and pipettes are available commercially. The device is inserted with the bitch standing on a table. There is normally no need to sedate

the bitch and most will tolerate vaginal insemination with minimal manual restraint.

After insertion, the device is advanced towards the base of the vagina being careful to avoid entering the urethra (the tube by which urine is evacuated from the bladder). Semen is then expelled into the anterior vagina as close as possible to the cervix. It is common practice to elevate the bitch's hindquarters for ten minutes after insemination to minimize the risk of semen being expelled.

Vaginal insemination is really only suitable when using fresh semen. Compared to intra-uterine methods, lower conception rates are achieved with chilled semen using vaginal insemination although the technique may still be successful and useful if there is nobody available who is skilled in transcervical insemination.

Uterine insemination

As previously stated, there are both non-surgical and surgical means of depositing semen directly into the uterus of the bitch. In the UK, Norway and Sweden ethical concerns for animal welfare discourage the use of surgical AI because non-surgical techniques are readily available and there is well-documented evidence of their success.

Non-surgical techniques

There are two techniques most commonly used to enable the non-surgical deposition of semen into the uterus. Individual inseminators tend to display a personal preference for using one or other of these transcervical techniques and both have proved successful when carried out by a person with the appropriate skills.

The 'Norwegian' technique utilizes a stainless steel catheter that is inserted through the cervix and into the uterus by means of a plastic guiding tube. The catheters are available in various sizes that are used as appropriate depending on the size of the bitch.

The guide tube serves to protect the catheter and to stretch the vagina without damaging the lining whilst the catheter is being inserted.

The Norwegian technique is simple and inexpensive. The inseminator must have the requisite skills to carry out the technique but these

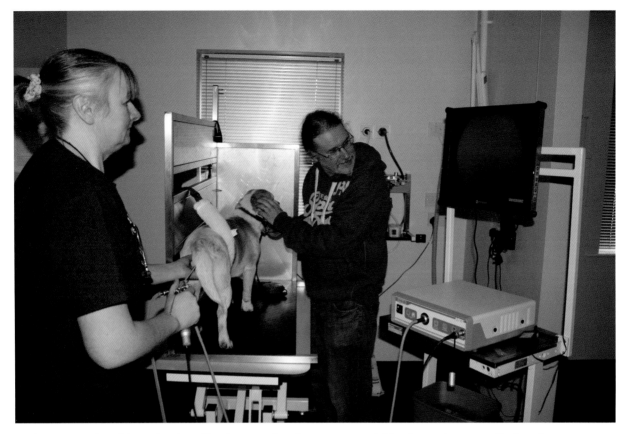

Endoscope-assisted insemination. The image taken by a camera within the endoscope, displayed on a screen, enables the inseminator to guide the catheter through the bitch's cervix immediately prior to insemination. (Photo: Louise McLean)

are easily taught and, with suitable practice, can be readily acquired.

The principal disadvantage of the technique is that the owner is unable to visualize the passage of the catheter into the uterus whereas the endoscope-assisted technique described below enables this to be demonstrated on a screen in association with the endoscopic equipment.

Endoscope-assisted transcervical insemination involves the use of a special, hollow, plastic tube within a rigid endoscope that is used to traverse the vagina and to help guide the tube through the cervix.

The endoscopic method requires expensive specialist equipment and the owner must attend a veterinary clinic or similar centre in order for the bitch to be inseminated. An advantage of the technique, however, is that it offers the owner convincing evidence that insemination has been successfully achieved because the whole process can be visualized via the screen associated with the endoscope.

Surgical insemination

Highest fertility rate and breeding success occurs when adequate semen can be placed at exactly the right time into the body of the anterior uterus. Intra-uterine deposition of semen can be accomplished using transcervical insemination and this technique is generally advised.

In circumstances where we are obliged to work with poor-quality semen or when there is an inadequate quantity of frozen semen available for transcervical insemination in order to achieve a valuable breeding, surgical insemination has been considered especially useful. It provides an optimum opportunity for successful pregnancy because success rates are generally excellent using this method, as it enables direct exposure of the semen to the developing egg.

To enable surgical insemination, however, the bitch has to be given a general anaesthetic and the surgical site aseptically prepared. An abdominal incision is made and the uterus is located. Semen is then directly injected into an anterior horn of the uterus via a small hypodermic needle. Only a single breeding can be performed and in order to optimize conception rates and litter sizes with a single insemination, accurate estimation of the time of ovulation and the corresponding timing of insemination is critical. A comprehensive pre-surgical examination and pre-anaesthetic screening are also advisable to ensure that the bitch is a good candidate for anaesthesia and surgery.

As the procedure requires general anaesthesia and abdominal surgery, ethical concerns for animal welfare discourage the use of surgical insemination. Not only is transcervical insemination regarded as the generally preferred technique in the UK but the Royal College of Veterinary Surgeons supporting guidance attached to the Code of Professional Conduct clarifies that UK animal welfare legislation (the Animal Welfare Act, 2006) prohibits canine surgical AI and as a consequence it is deemed a 'prohibited procedure'.

The Kennel Club in the UK has published policy on the use of AI and will refuse to register puppies born from the use of surgical insemination.

INDEX